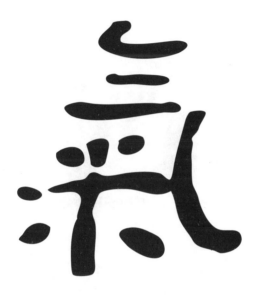

Ki (Chi) . . . *Life Force Energy*
Calligraphy by Masato Nakagawa

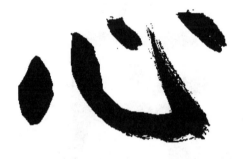

Kokoro . . . *Mind / Heart*
Calligraphy by Masahiro Oki

OVERCOMING CANCER

and Other Diseases in a Holistic Way

By

TOMEKO MITSUI

and Kazuko Tatsumura Hillyer, PhD

KOKORO PUBLISHING
NEW YORK

Gaia Holistic Inc.

d.b.a. Kokoro Publishing Company

20 West 64th Street, #24E

New York City NY 10023

Tel. No. (212) 799-9711

Fax. No. (212) 799-1661

Email: info@gaiahh.com

Overcoming Cancer & Other Diseases In a Holistic Way
© Tomeko Mitsui, and Kazuko Tatsumura Hillyer

Copyright © 2007
By Kazuko Tatsumura Hillyer

Printed in Canada

ISBN # 09704979-0-3

Designed by Dede Cummings and Carolyn Kasper / dcdesign

Cover art concept by Kazuko Tatsumura Hillyer
The cover design represents the planet earth ("Gaia"), with the top representing blue sky and sunlight, the middle section representing brown trees and the earth itself, and the red represenging the magma beneath the ground.
This edition is printed on acid-free paper that meets the American National Standards Institute z39.48 Standard.

Acknowledgements

My deepest appreciation to the following people in making this book a reality.

To my spiritual teachers: His Holiness the 14th Dalai Lama of Tibet, and Mother Theresa.

To my masters: Masahiro Oki, Masato Nakagawa, Osamu Tatsumura.

To Tomeko Mitsui for her tireless work in healing and writing the original of this book called "you can cure cancer with *ONNETSUKI*"

To Nicole who has given me much spiritual encouragement to do this book. When I met her she was diagnosed as "terminal" with only a few weeks to live, after exhausting all available cure of western medicine. After this *ONNETSUKI* treatment, she lived bravely two years more, even visiting Japan with me. She passed away in peace with stroke.

To Ms. Yukie Takagi and Mr. Masaru Shibuya of Mitsui Institute of *ONNETSU* Healing for their enormous support.

To Mr. Bunkichi Suzuki and IKKOSHA, the Japanese publisher of Tomeko Mitsui's book for their kind accommodation.

To Yoshiya Fujii for his knowledge of Far Infrared.

To Reiko Hillyer, Anna Borgmen de Martinez, Marie Sicari, Tashi Lama, Harriet Shields, Gil Padia and Dede Cummings for assisting me on the physical workings of this book.

Kazuko Tatsumura Hillyer

Warning – Disclaimer

This book is designed to provide information in regard to the subject matter covered. It is sold with the understanding that the publisher and the author are not engaged in professional services.

Every effort has been made to make this manual as complete and as accurate as possible. However, there may be mistakes both typographical and in content. Therefore, this text should be used only as a general guide and not as the ultimate source of information.

The purpose of this manual is to merely inform you of another knowledge which you might not have encounter. Otherwise, the author and KOKORO Publishing shall have neither liability nor responsibility to any person or entity with respect to any loss or damage caused, or alleged to be caused, directly or indirectly by the information contained in this book.

The ideas and suggestions contained in this book are not intended as a substitute for consulting with a physician. Always consult your doctor and other professionals.

If you do not wish to be bound by the above, you may return this book to the publisher for full refund.

Preface

WHEN YOU LOSE YOUR HEALTH, BECOMING ILL, especially with so called "incurable" or "difficult" diseases, you face the possibility of death. At this point, there are two paths in front of you. The first one is to say "why me" and blame everything around you, or refuse to see the truth, and only think that someone should help to heal you. You take for granted everyone's kindness as if you have the privilege or you "deserve" others' attention.

The second path is to say "why not me" and accept the possibility of this illness in you, to try to see the truth with open eyes, and to try to become the master of your own life and destiny.

These two paths are like a choice between sitting in the back seat of a car letting someone drive you OR sitting in the driver's seat. When you decide to sit in the driver's seat, you realize not only that you must choose the roads to take, the turns to make, but also you become aware of everything that is going on around you, and consequently you act according to the knowledge which you receive by being fully aware of everything.

Just as driving a car makes you aware of yourself, your action and your relationship to other factors/surroundings, so too can you become more aware of your own inner and outer body, physically or mentally. Then, this knowledge and increased awareness will inform you and help you to recognize what is going on in and out of yourself and help you to make the right choices and turns. When you begin to listen to your life-force, your own healing power will start working.

I decided to make this book available in English because it might help those who would like to choose the second path. Whatever choice you make and whatever result that choice might bring, the second path is to rely on your own healing power. Therefore there should be no regret. It is ultimately your responsibility for your own life force.

Chapter I is written by me as a sort of introduction to eastern modalities. Chapter II onwards is a free translation of Tomeko Mitsui's book of manual of **ONNETSUKI** method called "You can cure cancer with **ONNETSUKI**" published by IKKOSHA in Japan.

There are many holistic modalities available in the Orient. My wish is that more people might take the second path, by coming to know and experimenting with some of these rich modalities. I do not of course denounce western medicine but there are excellent benefits to eastern modalities which we should really look into. **ONNETSUKI** is one of those healing methods that has been remarkably successful in helping many people with serious conditions in Japan. I have experienced it myself. In the future, I intend to introduce more Japanese modalities which are producing exceptional results.

If this book can help even one person suffering with a serious illness, Mitsui & I shall be very happy. We have classes and treatments in New York. Please do not hesitate to contact us through mail, fax, or e-mail.

Gasshou

With deepest gratitude,
Kazuko Tatsumura Hillyer,

Contents

CHAPTER IV

CANCER THERAPY WITH *ONNETSUKI* FAR INFRARED HEAT

CHAPTER V

THERAPY FOR OTHER "DIFFICULT" DISEASES

CHAPTER VI
TESTIMONIALS

OVERCOMING

CANCER

*and Other Diseases
in a Holistic Way*

癌と散すにや
刀物はいらぬ
きれいな血液
流せばよい
トメ子

A scalpel is not necessary
for curing cancer.
Let the clean blood flow,
then, we can heal cancer.

— TOMEKO

THE WIND AND THE SUN

From the sky, the wind and the sun had a contest
to remove a man's coat.
The wind said, "I can take off the man's coat easily."
The wind started to blow hard on the man.
The more fiercely the wind blew,
the harder the man clutched onto his coat and did not let go.
The sun smiled,
and started to send the man warm, kind light.
Soon, the man felt very warm
and took off his coat by himself.

— THE PHILOSOPHY OF HOLISTIC HEALING

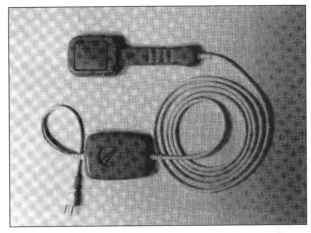

ONNETSUKI

Chapter 1

What Makes Us Heal Ourselves: "Ki" Energy

INCREDIBLE ADVANCES IN SCIENCE and medicine in the 20th century have brought us many ways to cure and heal illnesses, diseases and injuries. This has been a wonderful development for human kind. However, because of such vast knowledge and great excitement about new scientific discoveries and inventions, we have almost completely forgotten, or rather ignored, the other aspect of the healing process, which humans and all other living beings are given upon the birth on this planet. This is "Natural Healing Power". Before science was developed and medicine was invented by humans, we had the precious ability, instinctively or through experience, to fight against diseases and injuries. Through life experiences we knew how to heal injuries and diseases, what herbs or plants to take from nature for specific conditions, how to harmonize our life force energy with the healing energy of the universe, how to tune ourselves with our planet earth, how to exercise and stimulate our inner organs, how to breathe to take in maximum energy from the atmosphere, how to meditate to have our soul free of stress (harmful energy) and have a peaceful mind. We are born with the ability to heal any injuries or illness, from small to serious. So long as we are alive, our life force is constantly working for us to live in health and happiness. This is the Law of Nature. This LIFE FORCE energy is called *"KI"* in Japanese and "*Chi*" in Chinese.

As the last few hundred years have brought us so many amazing developments in science, medicine, we have totally forgotten this part of our ability. Now I think the time has come for us to recognize what we have forgotten and bring back some of this Natural Healing Power. It is my belief that in the next century, perhaps we will accomplish the glorious fusion of our scientific discoveries and developments with even more knowledge of Natural Healing Power in promoting our health and happiness. Already, many so-called "alternative medicines"—healing modalities, such as, Acupuncture, Herbal Medicine, REIKI, Taichi, Yoga, various heat treatments, mineral hot spring cure, Shiatsu, various massages, hand-on healing etc. have been widely experimented and gradually accepted in our society by us. But I think that the even more significant tendency is that we are beginning to realize the fact that a phenomenon called "*KI*" really EXISTS and CONTROLS our lives. We human do not only exist with the mechanics of our visible body but also we exist BECAUSE of "*KI*" life-force energy. Even scientists are now beginning to understand the importance of, or the quality of, the "*KI*" energy in maintaining and promoting our health, and are discovering the influences of "*KI*" energy in mental and physical well being.

Then what is this energy called "*KI*"? What is the "*KI*" in ourselves in relation to others and to the Planet in which we reside?

WHAT IS "*KI*"?

"*KI*" is as real as electricity, air, atmospheric pressure, temperature or gravity on the planet. "*KI*"(energy in our body and mind and as well as in space around us) is **The ultimate key to all of our health and happiness.**

1. "*KI* is the unseen force of nature that has infinite power and mysterious intentions. Every object on this planet carries "*KI*" which manifests in certain wavelengths.

2. "*KI*" in humans is an invisible light with a wavelength of

approximately 5 to 25 microns (similar to Far Infrared Ray of the sun light). This *"KI"* could sometimes show up in photograph.

3. *"KI"* runs in our body like an electric current. When this current is stagnated or clogged in the body, disorder can happen, which leads to illnesses. Keeping *"KI"* flowing smoothly throughout the body and organs working in harmony allows one to operate the body in good health and happiness as one harmonious integrated being.

4. In humans, there are numerous levels and kinds of *"KI"* just as there are numerous human beings. Some *"KI"* has consciousness and this consciousness will be either "positive" or "negative".

5. POSITIVE *"KI"* activates life force power, activates body and/or mind of humans or animals, and makes them lively, bright, positive, happy and healthy.

POSITIVE *"KI"* can heal or turn bad energy to good energy and promote a healthy life. When POSITIVE *KI"* is abundant and smoothly running through our bodies, we are healthy and happy. ***This is the force in harmony with the Law of Nature.***

NEGATIVE *"KI"* stagnates and causes illnesses, unhappiness, and even unfortunate incidents. NEGATIVE *"KI"* decreases the activities of living cells, dehydrates living organs, restrains the body or/mind and makes them pessimistic, and depressed. It degenerates cells, oppresses any activities of goodness. ***This is the force against the Law of Nature.***

It is interesting to note that, in Japanese the word (*Kanji*) for illness, "BYO**KI**", literally means "**KI** is sick", and good health is literally written as "GEN**KI**", which means that "**KI** is at its original (natural) state".

6. We can cultivate POSITIVE "**KI**" to the benefit of our lives by the following:

- By controlling our mind-attitude to be positive thinking at all times; by feeling full of thanks for all things, by caring for others, by looking at the bright side of all occurrences, and by avoiding a negative and critical mind.

- By re-supplying "**KI**" energy from the correct quality and amount of in-take (food, air, water etc) and eliminating unnecessary and harmful material, waste, and energy.

- By exercising the right amount and doing exercise which promote mindfulness, such as Taichi, Yoga, Meditation etc.

- By receiving "**KI**" energy directly from our universe and allowing "**KI**" to flow smoothly in our body. This can be assisted by many traditional or new holistic methods such as Far Infrared Sunlight, Tachyon energy, Magnets, SHIATSU hot springs treatments, herbal treatments, and various heat treatments.

Thanks to the recent scientific studies and reports, combined with traditional knowledge, we now know so much more about the relationship between health and universal energy. Among these Holistic modalities, this book is focused on the use of Far Infrared Sun energy. The research of usage of Far Infrared (FIR) has been much advanced in Japan and many products containing FIR are already produced. I dare say that use of FIR will be one of the most important medical developments of the 21st century. This book deals with one of the very successful applications of FIR on our body, which is already improving many illnesses and diseases.

WHAT IS FAR INFRARED?

- The daily sunlight we receive contains spectrums of different characteristics and effects according to its wave lengths.

- The wavelength of Infra Red spectrums are between that of microwave and that of visible ray (seven colors of rainbow).

- The wavelength of Infrared is 0.76-1000 microns and it occupies 80% of the sun's spectrum, covering a wide range. Infrared spectrums are classified into Near Infrared, Far Infrared (5-25microns), and Super Far Infrared.

WHAT IS THE CHARACTERISTIC OF FAR INFRARED?

- Far infrared is an invisible ray
- It is indispensable to any life on this planet. It has the ability to promote growth in animals and plants.
- It has the ability to penetrate deeply. It penetrates from inside of the object (interior to outside) and causes a heat deep within the object.
- It produces a natural and healthily comforting warm effect on the body. Upon application of the Far Infrared, the heat is felt much more mildly than other kinds of heat. The temperature does not rise too much.
- It is absorbed by many kinds of materials and then it

causes a heat deep within. As mentioned before, the wave-length of *"KI"* energy in our human body is 5-25 microns and wave-length of FIR is 8-15 microns. Therefore, FIR Ray occupies about 60% of the *"KI"* energy in our body. Within our body, *"KI"* energy and FIR Ray resonates and synchronizes in human cells. Therefore, FIR is very easily absorbed by the human body.

- Now then, what are the positive effects of Far Infrared on our body?

FAR INFRARED'S EFFECTS ON HUMAN BODY

- Rise of temperature in the depth of body

- Expansion of the capillary vessels

- Promotion of blood circulation

- Improvement of lymphatic disorder and an increase of the tissues' ability to regenerate.

- Positive effects on the control of abnormally excited sensory nerves and adjustment of function of the autonomic nerve system.

- Rejuvenation of human cells.

In the following chapters, we will introduce and explain a new device using of FIR energy *coupled* with heat called **ONNETSUKI** invented by Tomako Mitsui. This device is excellent, because FIR application is far better than other devices of physical therapies of the kind, such as Infra red heat, microwave method, hot packs, Moxa, carbon lamps etc. It also has ***absolutely no negative effect.*** Other heat treatments are directly transmitted only to the surface of the skin and feel very hot. This FIR device is not felt or sensed as strongly as others on our skin. If correctly used, this method will help many illnesses, and promote general health. It is our sincere hope that you elevate and nurture your own "Natural Healing Power" promotes your good *"KI"* with this device and accomplishes and maintains your health and happiness.

On the last words: I would like to say that all holistic healing modalities ultimately work toward the same goal; that is, to produce the positive *"KI"* and promote its smooth flow. On the contrary, western medicine often works against *"KI"* energy. Surgery cuts *"KI"* flow, and some aggressive medical methods disturb or weaken our *"KI"* energy.

In healing, the most important thing is the mind of thankfulness, gratefulness at every moments towards all occurrences around us: Toward air, food, family, friends. This humbleness brings enormous positive *"KI"* energy.

It is important to know these modalities bring much more results in helping ours, and others' Natural Healing Power when we apply them with positive, altruistic, caring heart. **At the end, the spirituality prevails. This positive *"ki"* is the key to all of our health and happiness.**

The word energy means life force (which can be interpreted as heat). All living things need this in order to survive. Energy is created in many ways. Some energy is created within us; other energy is taken from outside. Because energy is our life force itself, it promotes our blood flow, body fluid flow, and *"KI"* (life force) flow. It also changes food to the nutrients our body needs.

Supplying and promoting the flow of Ki energy and elimination: The mundane aspect

The word energy means life force (which can be interpreted as heat). All living things need this in order to survive. Energy is created in many ways. Some energy is created within us; other energy is taken from outside. Because energy is our life force itself, it promotes our blood flow, body fluid flow, and Ki (life force) flow. It also changes food to the nutrients our body needs.

WHEN OUR BODY TEMPERATURE FALLS, WE BECOME UNHEALTHY

In Japan and Asia, unlike in the U.S., inner body temperature is considered the key to health. We do everything we can to retain heat in our body. Today, inner body temperature tends to be lower than normal, causing imbalance and dis-ease. We have a traditional saying: "Upper cold, lower warm. Upper empty, lower solid." This means—contrary to what the Western world believes—that we should keep our feet and lower legs warm (especially the ankles), not the head or upper body.

RAISING OUR INNER BODY TEMPERATURE BY SUPPLYING HEAT FROM OUTSIDE THE BODY

A Japanese theory that has existed for thousands of years states that in order to be healthy, our inner body heat must be kept high. We believe that when the inner body temperature is low, cells are deprived of heat, which is energy, and that this prevents the cells and organs from functioning well.

Based on this theory, the Japanese have developed many methods for raising heat and body temperature in order to heat the body's deeper areas. It's interesting to learn that Dr. Abo recently explained this through his scientific discovery that "a person with low body temperature can't activate the lymphocytes in his white blood cells; therefore, his immune system can't function well, even if he has enough lymphocytes and white blood cells." This is why people with a low body temperature get sick easily.

- Low body temperature can be caused by:

- Lack of exercise.

- Excessive water intake. Asians view water intake quite differently from Westerners (especially Americans). We don't recommend taking in excess water, because we believe that doing so overworks and cools the kidneys and leads to bloating.

- Wrong food, wrong meal timing, irregular meal schedule.

- Stress, worry.

- Too many supplements, too much medicine.

- Smoking, and drinking too much coffee and soda.

- An irregular lifestyle, not enough sleep, late nights, late mornings.

Even if we're just sitting motionless, we're still creating heat in our bodies. Even when we're sedentary, our muscles produce more heat than any other part of our body—about 25 percent of our body heat. So as you can see, light exercise such as yoga, tai chi, and mindful walking are optimal.

ILLNESSES CAUSED BY LOW BODY TEMPERATURE

Low body temperature can cause a number of illnesses, including depression; bloating; swelling, women's problems, especially difficulties with menopause; headaches; dizziness; ringing in the ears; hair loss; age spots; wrinkles; aging skin; irritability; constipation; difficulties with urination; constant cold-like symptoms; cancer; diabetes; shoulder pain; lower back pain; ulcers; high blood pressure; infertility; diseases of the skin; collagen disease; multiple sclerosis; arthritis; rheumatism; prostate problems. Heating the body helps eliminate these illnesses.

A low inner-body temperature often accompanies symptoms of swelling, which in Asian diagnosis may be interpreted as a sign of illnesses. When your lower body swells in the afternoon, a heart problem is indicated. When your eyelids swell, there's a kidney problem. When your stomach is filled with water, there's a liver problem. It's important to determine and treat the root organs that are involved. But it's also important to warm our body in cases of general swelling, because swelling is a sign of toxic build-up. Warming the body increases blood flow to the kidneys, stimulating elimination.

The mundane aspects of receiving healing energy into our body can be accomplished in two ways:

1. Supplied from outside the body
2. Created within the body

Means to receive heat from outside the body

Far-infrared (sun-ray) therapy: The Mitsui Onnetsu method, using Onnetsuki (hand-held paddle)

Based on my many experiences of helping people heal themselves from simple back pain, neck pain, sports injuries, and even difficult and "incurable" diseases, I consider this therapy to be the crown jewel of Dr. Abo's theory. I am so grateful that he has explained the scientific reasoning that shows why the beliefs and methods we have practiced for thousands of years are correct and effective.

The principal theory of the Mitsui Onnetsu far-infrared method comes from an old Japanese belief that unhealthy body cells are deprived of heat and energy and are therefore cold—colder than healthy cells—and constantly shoot cold energy out from inside, toward the surface of the skin. In the Mitsui Onnetsu method, these cells are warmed with far-infrared rays that originate from the sun.

WHAT IS FAR-INFRARED?

In the late 1960s, NASA reported that rays of sunlight between 5 and 25 microns (or 8-14) are most beneficial to the growth of life. Light in this range promotes the life force, rejuvenates cells, and repairs damaged cells. These rays fall within the infrared range (.75 to 1,000 microns of wave length). Incredibly, the wave length of a healthy human body is also within this range. This fact helps explain the phenomenon of hand healing, or energy healing by touch.

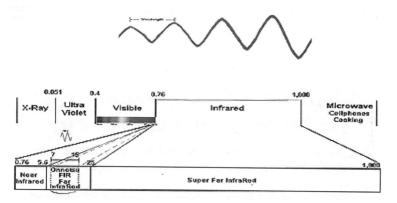

NASA's findings prompted a number of Japanese scientists to try to create tangible objects that would emit these kinds of rays constantly. After much research and experimenting, a number of scientists succeeded in creating objects composed of baked ceramic, various minerals, and stones. These baked ceramics were patented and developed into goods of many types. They were made into cotton and threads, and knitted into socks, shirts, and other types of clothing. They were made into mats, futons, and blankets. Healing lamps and other tools that emit rays in the far-infrared range of sunlight were created using these special ceramics.

WHAT IS ONNETSUKI?

Dr. Mitsui, an acupuncturist in her late seventies, had helped many people through traditional Japanese healing methods such as moxa, massage, and acupuncture. When she heard about far-infrared, she came up with an extraordinary idea: to combine the ancient theory of moxa with this newest technology of far-infrared. One characteristic of far-infrared is that the ray penetrates deep into the inner body from the surface of the skin—about 4 inches—reaching even to the organs. Dr. Mitsui believed that adding far-infrared ceramics to a heating mechanism would make a beneficial healing tool. In this way, Onnetsuki was born. The Onnetsuki is a handheld instrument that looks like a wand. It's remarkable in that it finds degenerated cells deep inside the body from the skin's surface. As I mentioned previously, the skin above these degenerated cells is cold. So when the Onnetsuki is placed on that part of the skin, the patient's reaction is hot, hotter than in other places. The practitioner then chooses to treat this spot until the reaction is consistent with that in other areas. It's also used to treat the spine and other parts of the body. So this new modality applies far-infrared to the body together with heat

Increase self-healing power (immunity) with
Far Infrared Onnetsu Therapy

THIS THERAPY is effective in improving all kinds of pains, chronic fatigue, diabetic, high blood pressure, rheumatism, stress, cancer etc. etc.

** Activating the cells by sending Far Infrared Energy heat with Onnetsuki **

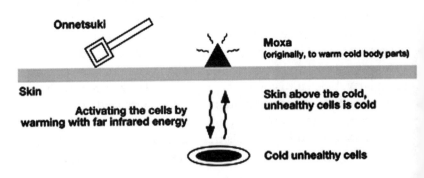

Onnetsuki

Moxa
(originally, to warm cold body parts)

Skin

Activating the cells by warming with far infrared energy

Skin above the cold, unhealthy cells is cold

Cold unhealthy cells

THE TWO PHASES OF FAR-INFRARED ONNETSU THERAPY

1. **Fundamental application:** The general promotion of one's healing power through the spine—the home of autonomic nervous system—which balances the sympathetic and parasympathetic nerves. According to Dr. Abo, this balance leads to the promotion of our immunity and self-healing power. Applying Onnetsuki to the spine and heating the spine area generates and improves the function of all the organs, including the heart, lungs, liver, gall bladder, kidney, bladder, spleen, stomach, pancreas, and large and small intestines. It also stimulates hormonal balance through the duodenum, thymus, and thyroid.

2. **Local application:** Once problematic spots are found, based on the patient's reaction to the Onnetsuki, far-infrared waves and heat are applied at those locations with the Onnetsuki. This rejuvenates the degenerated cells at these spots. Application of the Onnetsuki is repeated until the reaction subsides and the patient no longer feels hot in that area. This indicates that energy is reaching the cells, that the area and the degenerated cells are warming up, and that recovery has begun.

The Japanese people use this theory and have developed many methods for raising the body temperature and reaching deeper areas of the body.

Here is one example of how far-infrared Onnestu therapy works. This is the story of Lady "A." Her testimonial is at the end of this chapter (see page 221).

A lady came to our clinic in terrible condition at the final stage of brain cancer. She said that all her doctors had given up on her. She couldn't even walk, and her words were barely audible. Her right side, especially her arms and legs, were paralyzed. Her whole face and body was bloated. Her legs were very swollen, indicating kidney failure. I thought it would not be long before she left us, and that I could not possibly help her. So I asked her, "Are you ready to die?" She cried and said, "No, I'm scared." I explained that dying is not such a bad thing.

It's like changing old clothes for new ones. Your spirit will never die anyway, so don't fear death—simply be ready for it. Today you are alive, so make the best of it, without too much anxiety. Be positive that you'll live tomorrow as well, and the day after, and the day after, and so on… with full gratitude that you're alive.

We began daily Onnetsu therapy. Just one week later, on September 14, her blood test showed remarkable changes in the proportion of white cells (lymphocytes, macrophages, and granulocytes). By September 20 her blood test indicated further improvement in the lymphocytes. I was excited because this is almost exactly what Dr. Abo's theory indicates. Just as in Dr. Abo's explanation of the autonomic nervous system, the balance between her sympathetic and parasympathetic nerves had failed due to years of stress. Her sympathetic nerves were so overwhelmingly tense compared to her parasympathetic nerves that the proportion of her granulocytes had grown far too much in proportion to her lymphocytes, which were very weak.

White Blood Cell Differential	Healthy Person	Lady 'A' Aug 30, 2004	Lady 'A' Sep 14, 2004	Lady 'A' Sep 20, 2004
Lymphocite	35%	7.2%	22.4%	31.2%
Macrophage	5%	6.4%	10.4%	7.3%
Granulesite	60%	86.4%	67.3%	61.5%

I was amazed and encouraged, and realized that there was hope for her healing power! She came for treatments practically every day. Her language ability and use of her hands came back. The unhealthy hot spots disappeared from her head. Her appetite returned. Her recovery was remarkable in every aspect. By early 2005, she was cancer free!

The doctors were surprised. She lived very happily and healthfully for almost one year. She began traveling and enjoying life.

But her story doesn't end with this happy outcome. Unfortunately, about one year after her recovery, she felt so good and so healthy that she decided to go back to work as a day trader. She was excellent at day- trading, an extremely stressful type of trading in the stock market. Against my strong advice, she thought she would be all right. About six months later, her brain tumor reappeared, this time on the left side. This one grew very fast. When I learned of this recurrence, she was already in the hospital going through three Western treatments (radiation, chemotherapy, and surgery). I visited her, but a short while later she left us. We all have to go sometime, and this was her time. Everyday, I thank her for the great opportunity and the remarkable teaching she gave me.

Chapter 2

Overview of Far Infrared Heat Treatment

INTRODUCTION

MANY PEOPLE SUFFER FROM SO CALLED "incurable" diseases categorized as "*nambyo*" (incurable) by the Japanese government). Modern science has not been able to cure these diseases and we simply watch them get worse, especially in the case of cancer. These diseases cause stress in the entire family and depression in the patient facing death. Many of these patients visit my clinic one by one. They always say the same thing: "If only I had known about this therapy sooner."

I want to tell you about the wonders of Far Infrared energy coupled with heat (Far Infrared heat). This treatment does not require you to undergo test after painful test. You do not need surgery and you do not need to suffer side effects. This book introduces this method and serves as a manual for its use in diagnosis and self healing. I have provided numerous diagrams to further your understanding. Our clinic in Japan is also equipped with a facility dedicated to the study of this therapy. We are planning to expand internationally with an institute in New York.

No matter what, you must treat the parts of your body as precious. You have the power to repair any part of your body and keep it forever. Losing even one finger or a small part of one organ causes a great imbalance in body function. This means that other parts have to work harder to adapt. Each of the organs in our body has an important and distinct mission. They all work together. You must rid yourself of the idea that you can solve your problems by invasive procedures. For example, if cancer affects an organ, it may be that another organ has a problem that affects the cancerous one. It would be very damaging to cut out the cancerous organ and think all is well. The other organ will still have its affect and symptoms will not go away. You would have removed the cancerous organ for nothing.

Of course, I am not denouncing surgery. Sometimes you need it, but even if you think this is the case, you should always consult with a number of doctors. You should never simply listen to one doctor. People come to me who have had operations and then are told by their doctors that there is nothing more that can be done. Of course, it is difficult to treat someone like this. Try everything before you have an operation. To cut into the body is really to cut into one's life force, known as *"KI"* energy. Try to come to us and try the heat method first. This modality causes no harm and you can still choose to have surgery later. Hospital examinations and tests are so hard on the body. Using this Far Infrared heat machine (**ONNETSUKI**) in diagnosis not only does no damage, but also begins your own healing process. Your body will tell you what is wrong. Without fail, you can diagnose yourself and locate the problem. Your precious body is your own, and you must take care of yourself. You must live this philosophy. Try to use this book fully. I hope it will mean that at least one person will know one day earlier about the amazing effects of Far Infrared heat.

WHY FAR INFRARED HEAT
TREATMENT IS SO EFFECTIVE

We need heat in our body in order to live a healthy life. Of course, this sounds obvious. We take in air and food, and these elements, become heat or energy within our cells. Without this inner heat, the body does not function properly. It will be difficult to maintain a healthy body therefore illness results.

Consciously or unconsciously, we are constantly faced with physical and mental stress. This pressure accumulates gradually. Usually we think of stress in the context of a bad relationship or too much work. Stress, however, does not only accumulate during difficult times. Building a new house or getting married—seemingly good things—can be stressful because they involve changing one's lifestyle. This stress weakens the Autonomic Nervous System, which controls all body function.

Ninety percent of sickness comes from lack of inner heat caused by stress. If we can add heat or supplement the heat within the Autonomic Nervous System, we become very much like a plant after it has rained. As a plant recovers quickly from the drought, so our bodies recover from the lack of heat. Our circulation improves, and "*KI*" energy flows.

This treatment stimulates the Autonomic Nervous System by the application of Far Infrared heat to specific areas of the spine. No matter where the disease occurs, you must not forget to add heat to the Autonomic Nervous System. This therapy comes from Eastern medicine, not Western medicine.

My method of adding heat into a tired, rundown body is much more powerful than any diet or nutrition. There are no side effects and very immediate good effects. Circulation improves incredibly, giving your entire body oxygen. Residues are removed, and the cells come back to life so that they are able to fight disease. You also can slow down the aging process.

The chart below shows five people (A-E) before and after treatment. It analyzes the wavelengths of their energy (ideally 21 microns). After the treatment, people say that their body feels light and that they have more energy and appetite. Please note that even after one treatment,the wavelength measurement for each organ rises. When you are tired, this number declines rapidly, so you must continue to do this treatment.

Body wavelength analysis before and after treatment

	A		B		C		D		E	
	bef.	aft.	bef.	aft.	bef.	aft.	bef.	aft.	bef.	aft.
Immunity	2	10	9	16	16	17	6	15	11	17
Chest thymus	5	12	11	17	14	15	8	12	9	13
LIVER RELATED										
Liver	9	13	7	18	12	15	7	12	11	16
Gallbladder	8	11	7	12	14	16	7	15	8	13
Hypothalamus	4	12					8	15		
Sympathetic nerve	8	11	14	15	14	16	11	15	12	15
Parasympathetic	8	11	7	14	9	14	8	15	8	15
HEART RELATED										
Heart	10	14	15	17	11	14	9	16	11	15
Small intestine	7	15			13	16	9	15	11	11
Blood circulation	7	15	12	16			7	11	8	11
Arterial sclerosis					14	16				
SPLEEN RELATED										
Spleen	5	14	11	15	10	15	9	12	8	14
Pancreas	9	13			8	12	9	11	8	11
Diabetic					2	9				
Stomach	6	10	10	16	11	13	11	14	10	11
Thoracic nerve	6	14								
LUNG RELATED										
Lung	5	11	13	17	7	11	2	10	4	14
Bronchitis					8	12	7	13	8	12
Large intestine	6	11	12	16	11	14	8	15		
Stress			6	12			7	12		
KIDNEY RELATED										
Kidney	8	15	9	17	8	12	7	11	7	15
Thyroid			4	10			6	11	7	12
ADDITIONAL										
Respiratory ctr.							6	11		
Cancer	9	14					9	11		

ONNETSUKI itself looks like nothing. People want to believe only in large, contemporary facilities and impressive, complicated machinery of modern hospitals. They rely on doctors who can only operate under these conditions. People question whether such a little, inexpensive-looking machine can help. Don't forget, though, that there are no side effects. Before you go to the hospital for invasive procedures, please try this. You have nothing to lose. Many people give up and die after believing only in conventional medicine. For them, every day counts. I sincerely hope you try this method. The first step is to stop believing that any disease is incurable or fatal. As long as you have hair and nails that grow, you have plenty of healing power within you.

FEATURES OF FAR INFRARED TREATMENT BY *ONNETSUKI*

- It has a good effect on 90 percent of disease and never has a bad effect.

- From the surface skin, one can detect the body's inner health. *ONNETSUKI* is as good or even better than X-rays, endoscopes, etc. If you go to the hospital, the tests themselves are very tiring, painful and burdensome to an already sick body. Furthermore, they don't even begin the healing process.

- No matter where the illness occurs, *ONNETSUKI* detects it effectively. Depending on how your skin reacts to heat, you can diagnose the functional ability of the head, stomach, lungs, nervous system, muscles, etc. In only 30 minutes, one can diagnose anything unusual from head to toe.

- *ONNETSUKI* can detect an illness or unusual development before it would be found by a conventional examination and even before you are aware of its symptoms.

With this machine, one can accomplish detailed EXAM-INATION, EARLY DIAGNOSIS and SELF HEALING at the same time. Patients who otherwise would have died can regain health with *ONNETSUKI*. So called "incurable" diseases, such as diabetes, cancer and rheumatoid arthritis, are those that respond best to this treatment.

PREVENTING CANCER

Heat treatments can help prevent cancer. No one wants to get cancer, but cancer can be developing within the body without our knowledge or consciousness. It is even developing within the seemingly healthy body. Cancer takes a long, long time to develop. By the time cancer is detected by X-ray, it already has progressed and often is in the end stage. When cancer is found, the first reaction is often to recommend surgery. By this time, though, the cancer already has spread throughout the body. Thus surgery is not necessarily helpful. Doctors recommend early surgery saying that it prevents cancer from spreading. This is a wrong concept in my opinion. It is like cutting off the top of a mountain thinking the top was all that there was. This is because western medicine has no way to detect beneath the surface and doctors might not realize the entire body is already affected.

But there is a way. Use **ONNETSUKI**. It is a detector with super ability. Perhaps you cannot imagine how you, from the surface of skin, can learn what is happening inside your body. You can pinpoint the location of any irregularities inside the brain, internal organs, bones, muscles, and soft tissue. And you can self-heal by applying heat. It doesn't take more than 30 minutes, to examine and it's very, very simple. It provides immediate diagnosis and can start immediate healing. It has no side effects. It is like magic.

You can even detect brand-new cancer cells and quickly make them disappear. It is like cutting off a new bud before it becomes a growing flower. You can extinguish the fire before it begins to rage. When searching with **ONNETSUKI**, the patient notes a sharp heat reaction on the skin (hot spot). This hot spot reveals the seed of the illness. You can apply more heat in this area to prevent or stop progress of disease. In case of cancer, this hot spot feels as a, sharp pain. Cancer is affecting more and more people of younger age. Please do not think that because you're young and healthy that you are cancer free. All people who have stress have the potential to become cancer patients. For those who have much stress, it is very easy to get cancer. If you wish, you can prevent cancer by using *ONNETSUKI* as a detector. For those young people, the cancer progress is very fast. The cancer is usually much more rigorous and vicious, so you must take care of it immediately. Don't wait. By the time cancer is detected by modern medicine, it is in the whole body. Therefore, even if you have an operation, it will occur somewhere else in a few years. *ONNETSUKI* is also very good for maintenance of general health.

Cancer is a disease of the entire body, not individual body parts— even if you surgically remove it will emerge in another location. I am very sorry to hear that so many people die because they do not realize this fact. Illustrated in this chart are various disease steps. In Steps 1,2,3 the body is really easily restored to normal and a healthy body. *ONNETSUKI* can detect cancer from step 1, but western medicine can not detect cancer from step 1. Western diagnosis can perhaps find cancer only around step 3 or 4. When you develop a cancer up to step 4, it is difficult but still possible to bring back to step 1 by *ONNETSUKI*. Cancer begins showing up on X-rays at step 4or 5. Step 6 is already too late. You have no awareness of cancer yourself in the first 5 steps. You think you are healthy, and by the time it is detected by western medicines, it is too late. When you go to the hospital, they offer you **the three therapies—*surgery, chemotherapy,* and *radiotherapy.*** Those methods are really robbing your body's life force. The cancer cells might get weaker, but the body becomes so weak that it is often not able to cope with the procedures. Cutting the cancer out is not going to be good enough. However, cancer is not something to be afraid of if you can find it and prevent it early on. X-rays find cancer too late and operations do not cure the disease at that stage. However, if you can insert heat in the right places—any hot spots or sharp pain spot you detect with **ONNETSUKI**—and restore them back to step 1, cancer will not develop. In this method, the largest organ of the body, the skin, is used to detect inner organ abnormalities. This is a mysterious power of the skin—it has a close relationship to inner organs. It is a mistake to ignore this important relationship. In the final stages, Western medicine and doctors tells you that you are hopeless and give you generally how long you'll live. You think your only hope is to rely on a doctor. But you should not rely only on a doctor. You must rely on yourself and your own healing power. Often people die simply because they do not take actions on their own, believing only the date of the death that doctor gives you. The stress caused by this declaration is enormous and more harmful than ever. Cancer is not incurable. This is a false myth. One can fight back against cancer.

ARE YOU TREATING THE WRONG AREA IN THE WRONG WAY?

Some diseases cannot be diagnosed by modern technology, and we cannot cure with anything when we do not know its cause. In Japan, the government classifies these diseases as "nambyo" or "difficult/incurable."

These include, but are not limited to, Parkinson's disease, Meniere's disease, Raynaud's disease, Tourette's syndrome, Multiple sclerosis, and Collagen Vascular disease. Western medicine looks at the body part in isolation and tries to remove the symptoms only, thereby, sometimes missing the right area to treat in the right way. On the contrary, with the **ONNETSUKI** therapy, these "difficult" diseases are not that baffling.

This therapy is quite effective on these diseases that are considered to be "incurable," because it recognizes the treatment point which is not necessarily where the symptom manifests. For example, Meniere's disease is generally considered a disease of the organs of the ear because it leads to deafness and vertigo. Doctors usually treat the ear only. I believe it to be a dysfunction of the thyroid gland due to stress. If you keep treating only the ear, it is never going to be healed. I have successfully treated this in two-three sessions. Diabetes is caused by a hormonal imbalance due to stress. The usual treatment is to adjust the diet. At the present time, Western medicine is focused on curing the symptoms with insulin. You can greatly improve diabetes by restoring hormonal balance with **ONNETSUKI**. Because this disease is due to stress-induced hormonal imbalance, it can recur if there is a recurrence of stress. Raynaud's disease is also caused by stress, which leads to an abnormality in the sympathetic nervous system. In some of the most severe cases, the legs must be amputated. Applying heat along the spine is very effective. This is a difficult disease because usually the wrong location is being treated.

The wrong treatment in the wrong area can occur even on a simple case such as the pain on upper stomach, or lower rib cage. Sometimes, one misdiagnoses this as a stomach problem and keeps taking medicine for it. This can be a case of Intercoastral Nerve pain and if treated as such by **ONNETSUKI**, the pain can disappear easily.

BEFORE YOU DELUGE YOUR BODY WITH LOTS OF MEDICINES

You should not have to take very much medicine. A very, very small amount can be effective. But if you go to a doctor, you are given so many different medicines—sometimes an entire bag full! The medicine, even if it is good, loses its effectiveness if you take it all the time as your body develops the immunity to the medicine. Your body also reacts to medicine by trying to get rid of the toxins in it. The kidneys and liver especially become very over-worked and exhausted. The side effects may really hurt the liver, but even "good" medicine gradually has a negative effect. The doctor says, "Drink this. Take this and this and this." Because you believe in your doctor and obey his orders blindly, your inner organs fail. Your natural system of fighting loses power because your body is artificially supported by the medicine, and gradually your body becomes very weak.

I am not saying that you should not take medicine, but don't rely on medicine blindly. You quickly diminish your own healing power with which you were born, which you were given by God. Your whole body begins to rely on taking medicine and becomes lazy. With you body's healing power so weak, any disease cells love to grow and begin taking over. In order to increase your own healing power, you have to make your own healing power healthy and strong.

Take, for example, medicine to reduce blood pressure. They say that if you start taking it, you have to take it all your life. This shows how bad it is. If you have to take it all you life, it is not a good medicine. I also question taking blood pressure just one time only and in one body location. To consider this the result for the entire body does not make sense to me. The general population is so varied: small people, big people, thin people, fat people. The environment is different around the world. The temperature is varied. Everything is different. The conditions of each person, each day, are different. We are living with variable blood pressure. To establish one set of standards seems strange to me. Is it really correct to say that because your blood pressure does not meet Western standards that you must take this medicine all your life?

Some people have diet particulars. Some people may wear habitually corsets or tight brassieres. Also, some people are very tense in a doctor's office and can make their blood pressure rise. Without taking all these things into account, one just measures blood pressure at the arm and decides that it is high or low. Ideally, blood pressure should be measured not just one time in one spot but at different times and in different parts of the body. You should take measurements this way for several times at different time of the days, when you are healthy and know your own normal blood pressures. That should be the natural way.

Human beings walk and stand on two legs. Therefore, naturally blood pools in the legs and when blood pressure decreases the blood that reaches the brain may decrease. After a long time, the brain is poorly nourished and its function may diminish. The number of brain cells decreases and they do not recycle properly. Then you begin to lose mental sharpness. Even if you take medicine, it will not remedy this situation. In fact the person who habitually takes more medicines for long time, faster the sharpness of brain goes.

There are so many diseases in the world that one cannot cure by Western methods. If you go to doctors with these diseases, they keep giving you pills. All this medicine has side effects, and some may be toxic. Doctors give you more pills to cure the side effects caused by the medicine given earlier sometime it goes on and on like this. The doctor says that if you don't take this you will die, so you keep taking it. This is a vicious cycle. When you get older, hardening of the arteries is a natural phenomenon but you should still not try to control blood pressure only with medicine because there may be another reason that you have high, or low, pressure. The secret of long life is in taking the least amount of pills possible.

Rheumatoid arthritis is caused by an imbalance of the Autonomic Nervous System, which results in hormonal imbalance. If you apply heat and balance the Autonomic Nervous System, it often improves. However, if you are taking all the medicines prescribed, it becomes difficult to cure even with this heat treatment.

DON'T LOSE YOUR LIFE BY MISDIAGNOSIS

Sometimes, contemporary medicine misdiagnoses illnesses. One lady had a headache and went for tests. They told her she had lung cancer and a brain tumor. Her entire family was depressed. So many tests, painful tests, were done, without a definite diagnosis. They recommended brain surgery. When I checked her, there was no reaction indicating cancer in either the lung or brain. The headache was simply caused by trigeminal nerve pain. It ceased after I treated her. Whether or not the expensive CT scanner was broken or the technician lacked knowledge, she was about to have surgery and all sorts of other treatments. She would have died.

An 84-year old woman was diagnosed with cancer affecting two-thirds of her left lung. I checked her out, and there was no reaction of cancer in that area. She had taken very strong medicines that caused side effects, including brittle bones and the inability to fight off germs.

So many people have said they have cancer, but I think people often die or are dying because they are misdiagnosed. With depression, stress and all these cancer treatments, some people die. So please, guard your life. It is so complacent to leave it up to the doctor, and it is very wrong. You have to guard your own body. If you remove the lung, part or whole, it cannot grow back. Try all other methods before you agree to do that. There is no organ that is not necessary in our body. Each has important functions. All organs function together and balance each other. Do not casually treat individual parts of your body. Do not causally undergo surgery.

A 49-year-old male experiences abnormal, uncoordinated body movement and became weaker and weaker. In the hospital, he was diagnosed with a brain abnormality in the cerebellum. They said he would live no longer than five years. When I treated him the fourth time, he began to move more normally. I told him that his nervous system, which had been damaged by medicine, would gradually become well. His face lit up and his life force returned. He was very happy to have such strong energy, especially because he had been told he would die.

Another man had pain in the left abdominal area. In the hospital, they could not find the cause. They kept giving him morphine to subdue the pain. Soon, the morphine became ineffective and the pain was excruciating throughout the day and night. When I examined him, I found that duodenal inflammation was preventing the pancreatic juice from flowing normally. I treated the duodenum, opened the duodenal passage, and the pain immediately went away. If they had kept using morphine without finding the cause of his pain, the pancreas would have digested itself with its own juice.

At my institute, I have discovered a number of misdiagnoses. If something had not been done, all theses patients would have died. There are many such examples. Many people are being misdiagnosed at the hospital. You are responsible for your life, whether you live or not depends on you alone. No matter how authoritative the hospital seems, it might sometimes be wrong for you. Check yourself out more than one place.

With **ONNETSUKI**, you can examine the body completely without the risk of misdiagnosis. Your reaction is very accurate no matter where the illness or abnormalities occur. Even an amateur can understand **ONNETSUKI** reaction. You also can tell whether or not you have cancer. Your body will tell you, before it can be detected clinically. Remember chemotherapy, operations, and testing beats up and tires the body. You may not have to go through this. You can diagnose yourself by diligently checking your body with **ONNETSUKI**. I want you to learn this method. Of course, the fact whether or not you will be successful depends a great deal on your ability. There are people who can teach you. If you have applied **ONNETSUKI** and you experience a sharp, stabbing pain, there is an element of cancer in the area. By repeating the heat application, this sharp pain reaction becomes weaker and more tolerable. If the heat is tolerable and feels good, then the illness is on the way to recovery.

Why do so many people come to me? People who come to me have been abandoned and rejected by traditional practitioners. I wish there were more people that came to me at the beginning because it would be so much easier and faster to return their health. Many of my patients come very late when there is no way to help. So many diseases can be helped. All you have to do is diagnose your reaction to **ONNETSUKI** and apply the heat to the right places.

༺

Chapter 3

Challenging the Cancer

WHAT CAUSES CANCER?

OUR BODY HAS A NUMBER OF STREAMS, including blood, hormones and heat. All these flow smoothly when one is healthy. When you take in food, it goes through the digestive tract and leaves the body. That also is a stream. There are several currents of heat in the body. Water goes through the body and comes out as urine. All of these streams should flow normally.

With stress, some of the streams become unbalanced or clogged. When you have clean blood, smoothly flowing throughout your body, giving your body nourishment and oxygen and taking away the residues, you are healthy. However, our complicated society today causes great physical and mental stress. It is too powerful. Our life force is so threatened by that the Autonomic Nervous System becomes unbalanced. We therefore cannot maintain a normal life force flow and we become ill. Cancer is no exception to this.

Before we discuss the elements that cause cancer or how to fight them, we must think about what happens with an accumulation of stress. When stress increases adrenal hormones are over-released. This causes adrenal gland weakness that affects the immune system. When immunity is low, the entire body becomes susceptible to illness. Cancer does not arise outside your body. You cultivate it for a long time—for months and years. When cancer cells are formed, your natural healing system will work against cancer. But when your killer cells are weak, they cannot fight against the cancer. Cancer occurs:

- in organs that are not very active
- in areas that do not receive oxygen or nourishment because of poor circulation
- in areas where blood stagnates
- with pH imbalance in body fluid
- in organs that are abused
- by toxic side effects of medicine
- by the overuse of medicine.

When the Autonomic Nervous System is unbalanced, energy is lacking. The cancer sometimes shows up in one place, but by that time cancer cells have spread throughout the body. These cells are waiting to grow. Cancer does not jump from location to location like the pollination process. This is why surgery of the affected areas does not prevent recurrence. The cancer is very deep and rooted. Without your awareness the cancer was growing for years and years. By the time, you recognize cancer, the entire body is affected by cancer. Many people have no complaints on regular physical examinations for years but actually have cancer.

MODERN MEDICINE'S APPROACH TO TREATING CANCER

One should not be so frightened of cancer. Modern science says that cancer is an incurable disease. They say that much progress has been made, but it's simply untrue. They still use three basic treatment methods—surgery, radiation, and chemotherapy. Cutting out cancer, burning it with radiotherapy, or killing it with chemotherapy are only means of dealing with it superficially without finding the root to the cause. Modern medicine does not take any responsibility for the eventual death after these treatments. Cancer cells do not die as easily as normal cells. They are very, very strong and strange. Unless you really diligently work on them, they will come back very quickly. For example, the treatment of melanoma is surgery and radiation. It will recur. Using my treatment, it is cured and rarely recurs. If you see a black beauty mark around the chest, back of the neck, or middle back, you have to be very careful and watch it. If you apply **ONNETSUKI**, and you have cancer, you will feel unbelievable stabbing pain.

If you know the root of cancer, treatment is easy. Common culprits are food, cigarettes, etc. Of course, smokers have a greater risk or getting cancer than non-smokers, but this is not the only factor involved.

Comments on the three basic cancer treatments:

1. Operating disturbs the flow of "**KI**" energy in our body and works against healthy life force. When cancer shows up again, it is removed surgically again. Gradually, more and more of the body are cut out. Sometimes, doctors remove lymph nodes. This is very, very dangerous. Lymph nodes are our partner in fighting cancer. It is not wise to remove them.

2. With chemotherapy, you lose hair, vomit and feel crazy. These drugs may or may not kill cancer cells, but they definitely damage and kill normal cells.

3. Radiation is considered a cancer-causing agent and yet it is being used in the treatment of cancer.

In my opinion, it is unbelievable to call these the "three best cancer therapies." These three treatments further damage a body already weakened by cancer. We cannot live fully and fight the disease.

WHY WE SUPPOSEDLY CANNOT CURE CANCER

1. Because the cause of cancer is not known and we are, therefore, working in darkness.
2. The clinical diagnosis of cancer is too late. When it has progressed too far, the body is very weak and does not have much power to fight.

3. The present methods of cancer healing are inadequate. Cancer is a disease of the entire body. Cutting one part out does not help. Removing important organs causes an imbalance in the body causing the body to become weak thereby allowing cancer to spread rapidly. Chemotherapy has strong, toxic side effects and kills healthy cells. The degree of damage done to healthy cells is unknown or unexplained. People, who undergo chemotherapy often spit up blood, suffer damage to their inner organs and lose their hair. If a chemotherapy agent touches the skin, the skin dies immediately. The liver can fail. Radiotherapy is like putting an atomic bomb into your body. We worry about atomic tests all over the world, but we are using the same energy in medicine. I cannot imagine why this is done. It might stop cancer from growing, but it does not kill the cancer.

4. Doctors say cancer has spread to another location in the body. It is not unusual to have cancer in any part of the body. If you have cancer in one location, it will most likely emerge in another. This is why we cannot simply operate and think cancer is eliminated.

5. Lymph nodes enlarge for two reasons—because lymph nodes themselves are cancerous, and/or because they are inflamed (fighting off the cancer's infection). When you have an infection, lymph nodes increase in size. Why, without even examining, are they removed? This is wrong.

6. Psychologically, you give up because you think that cancer is incurable. You think cancer is a death sentence.

7. All of the tests and examinations are very harmful to the body. Doctors take out blood, put in medicine, insert cameras, remove body parts surgically, etc. All of this makes the body weak, including and especially certain substances you need to take in order to have the tests are often harmful.

8. The examination is not 100 percent thorough. Sometimes through examination you can only find the cancer in one spot. Often other locations are overlooked. You have to work with different specialists and go from doc-

tor to doctor, hospital to hospital. You have to go through the same routine of horrible testing again and again.

9. After a cancer operation, living five years is considered a great success. Three-year survival rates for gastrointestinal cancer are about 50 percent, liver cancer 12 percent, lung cancer 19 percent. Even if you survive, you have to deal with complications, lifestyle adjustments, and possible handicaps.

10. People give up because they think there is nothing they can do except die. Often, doctors tell these people that they will die in a certain period of time. These people take this information as absolute truth. They are letting the doctor do everything and think they have no choice and nothing to say or do that matters.

11. Doctors who treat cancer may say that if you don't agree to surgery right away that you won't live for very long. The patient becomes deeply depressed. Who is a doctor to say that one has three months to live? Patients believe this!

12. Cancer is often misdiagnosed. Basic diagnosis is done by detailed, advanced machinery. However, often one doctor says it is cancer and another may not. Sometimes doctors' opinions conflict. You think the machine is foolproof, but it is inaccurate at times. I have tested several patients who had been misdiagnosed prior to coming to me:

A 70-year-old woman went to the doctor saying that she had a headache and was told she had a tumor. The doctor said they could not operate but would administer chemotherapy. Once she started chemotherapy, she completely lost her appetite and energy. I diagnosed her only with nerve pain. It disappeared after two **ONNETSUKI** treatments.

Another example. A 50-year-old woman who had been told her entire body was full of cancer and that she had only two months to live. She had had one breast removed. Because she was coughing, the doctor told her that the cancer must have migrated to the lung. They believed her brain and three areas of bone were also involved. She took chemotherapy for three years. I examined her and did not believe she had any cancer. I asked her to stop the chemotherapy. I used **ONNETSUKI** and within three weeks, she became very strong. Her husband was so surprised when he visited her. Everybody was very surprised. Of course, because there was no cancer, the treatment worked very well. She did not have cancer at that time. And she was undergoing chemotherapy. No wonder she had very weak bones and a terribly weak body. Two weeks later, she neglected heat treatments, thinking she was already well. She became very weak and returned to the same hospital. They told her that she was weak because she stopped the chemotherapy. They restarted the treatment and she became weaker and weaker until she eventually died.

A 55-year-old man was diagnosed with lung cancer and came to me. **ONNETSUKI** elicited a reaction, but it was not that of cancer. I suggested that he go to another hospital for a second opinion before he was mistakenly treated for cancer. This man, however, listened to a relative who said that the hospital was the best hospital with the best doctors and there was no way that he could have been misdiagnosed. The doctor at the hospital said that the cancer was in the very end stage and that he could not operate. Within 24 hours, he started chemotherapy. The patient experienced so much pain and suffering that he finally sought a second opinion in another hospital, which was the same as mine. No cancer. With my heat treatment, he became well again and left the hospital.

13. Young people have bodies and minds that are very rundown and weak. In the past, a family had many children who became very strong, with a strong life force. They fought each other, they helped each other and they raised each other. In modern times, families have only one or two children, and they are overprotected and cared for too much, so that they have weak bodies and minds. At the same time, parents are eager for them to

get high grades and force them to study, adding a lot of stress. When they finally go out into society, they are faced with other pressures, tremendous pressures of doing well, that further stress the body and mind. So more young people get cancer nowadays. Cancer is diagnosed in younger and younger patients. Today, people in their 20-40's get cancer. The disease progresses quickly in the young. In these cases, the root of the cancer was probably already present in middle school or high school. Therefore, soon after entering society, they get cancer. Then, as soon as you are diagnosed, you get an operation. If you don't, the doctors will tell you that you will die and it will be too late. There is no thought of educating in the Alternative Methods. The doctor is a human being and is neither Buddha nor God, and so, of course, they sometimes give the wrong advice. The most important thing to provide is good guidance so that people can make his or her own decisions. It is cavalier to off the conveyor belt-style of treatment consisting of operation, chemotherapy and radiation. That should not be the only way to advise the patient.

CHALLENGING CANCER WITH *ONNETSUKI*

The genes with which a person is born are impossible to change and therefore the best way to avoid getting cancer is to eliminate stress. This means that one should strive daily to balance the Autonomic Nervous System. **ONNETSUKI** is amazingly effective at balancing the Autonomic Nervous System by adding energy to one's life force. I believe that if stress and certain inherited genes do not come together, cancer does not start. This is not just true for cancer but also for other illnesses. In order to prevent sickness, you must take away the stress daily by providing your body with heat and energy. If you do this, you can prevent disease.

The basic healing method of **ONNETSUKI** is to apply heat to the entire spine and back. After that, you apply heat to the area where the patient feels heat on the skin. The degree of heat corresponds to the severity of illness. You will be surprised at how fast the illness improves. The Far Infrared heat penetrates all the way through into your inner organs without scarring the body. Without fail, **ONNETSUKI** reveals any disorders or unusual activity of the inner organs. More complicated tests are not necessary. If cancer is present, the patient does not feel heat, but notes a strong pain, similar to being stabbed with a knife. Although the pain is very intense, it quickly disappears, especially if it is in the beginning stage. Because cancer reacts to heat so quickly, I think it is, in a way, obedient.

Do you know the story of the wind and the sun? The sun and the wind had contest to remove a man's coat. The wind blew like crazy to try to remove a man's coat. The man clutched his coat even tighter. The sun came out, and the person took off his coat by himself. This is a very good example of cancer treatment. Instead of attacking and killing that makes the cancer even stronger, let us use positive treatment—helping the cancer leave on its own.

Cancer does not emerge suddenly in one spot. It develops over a long, long time. The body itself becomes a type of cancer. The roots are there and all over the place; deep roots that emerge as a bud here and there. Modern medicine says it has spread and is jumping. This is incorrect. No matter how much you cut into a body to remove the cancer, you can not eliminate it. You may heal after surgery, but this is because your own healing power was still strong, not because the cancerous area was removed. Until one accepts this idea, the cancer is going to come out again. Then, It will then be labeled "incurable".

Cancer has been caused by stress. Today's cancer treatment is like pushing a deeply depressed person off the cliff when they are trying to commit suicide. And, on top of this, chemotherapy is used to kill the cancer cells. Cancer cells, however, are very, very strong—much stronger than normal cells. Therefore, normal cells die faster than cancer cells. Radiation is considered to cause cancer, but why is it used as cancer treatment? A healthy person exposed to radiation can die within two or three years. The doctor says that radiation stops the progress of cancer. That might be true, but here again, I think that your own healing power is at work while your life force is still strong. It is said that surgery, chemotherapy, and radiation therapy work in the early stages. This may be because they only provide a trigger for our fighting cells. The same trigger can be given by heat treatments with

ONNETSUKI.

A medical book I read says that cancer is carried by the blood from one part of the body to another. This does not make sense to me. If a cell leaves a part of the body, then it is dead. The body eliminates it. Whey does one think that cancer cells are different from other cells? Why does it leave one place and then start growing in another? This happens because at the ground level it is all connected. This ground is the body infected with cancer cells. Cancer cells bud from the ground at its roots and don't spread form bud to bud. So if what I have said is correct, one can work to change it. If the bloodstream is turbulent, it should be restored to smooth flow. If the organs are not very active, then one should give energy to rejuvenate the systems that became old. If you accept this philosophy, then cancer cells will gradually be conquered by normal cells. Cancer is not a monster anymore.

If you think there is no other method of dealing with cancer, please try this, ***ONNETSUKI.*** Depending on how you do it, it is amazing. Some cancers go away very quickly. Do not believe that the only and best way to cure the cancer is to operate. Why don't we try this method first before any other method? It's not too late. Do not think of surgery from the beginning. A part that is cut will not grow back. Cancer can be conquered by this method, but after you have surgery, it will be difficult because the body will be weakened by the trauma of surgery. No matter how many places cancer is growing, I can assure you that one can be helped before resorting to surgery. Of course, if you have progressed to the end stage, it is difficult to save you even with ***ONNETSUKI.***

Please know that what modern medicine refers to as the beginning stage is already cancer in the last stage. You have it throughout your system, and your body is very weak. Cancer is not a contagious virus from the outside environment. It does not arise externally. It is a cancer susceptibility that you created habitually. When you are diagnosed with cancer, you have been cultivating cancer for at least 10 years. It grows so gradually at the beginning.

Curing cancer is not a miracle. The world does not recognize cancer unless a doctor has diagnosed you. But when I help someone with a diagnosed cancer by a respected hospital recover, they say that perhaps the diagnosis was wrong. They say cancer cannot be so simple to cure. If they learn that such a small little machine can cure cancer, of course, the hospital will have problems when they are charging so much money for their famous three treatments. If I have helped so many cancer patients, I'm sure that many other people can do it. Please, I am so troubled by the present situation: immediately after diagnosing cancer follows test after test after test and only a menu with three options is provided for treatment. They say that having a longer life is a miracle. This philosophy is wrong. So long as we live, we have our own life force. We need to help our life force conquer because our life force always wants to live. We have our own "Natural Healing Power", we have to find a way to stimulate this.

Hospitals and doctors take such a cavalier approach to cancer patients' dying by declaring that there is only a certain time left to live. This death sentence deeply affects patients mentally and physically, which is a blow to an already weakened body. If they do not believe they can cure, why do they do all these things? I have made very strong statements without inhibition, but in my experience, I can say that I can improve cancer in 80 percent of cases up to the third stage. At the very last stage, when the tissues are dead, and especially if the patient has lost hope of living, I cannot help. Of course, one should do this treatment as quickly as possible, but it is more difficult to help the longer the delay. There are no side effects associated with this treatment. Heat weakens cancer cells. Researchers are looking into how to put heat into organs. Contemporary medicine is looking into it. However, this little machine puts Far Infrared heat deep into the organs. Then you can begin to use your own healing power, your own immune system, and your own killer cells. Bit by bit, you become stronger. Lymph nodes and macrophages are our friendly killers and cleaners, which attack cancer cells and conquer them. The hospital method of three treatments, in a way, works against what I am trying to do by weakening one's own healing power.

Finally, I can't stress enough the importance of mental attitude in one's recovery. The patient must have a strong will to live. By reducing the pain and suffering while treating cancer, the Far Infrared heat method promotes a feeling of well being and the will to live.

Chapter 4

Cancer Treatment with Onnetsuki *Far Infrared Heat*

ADVICE

IF YOU ARE DOING THIS METHOD at the same time as hospital treatments, it will have no effect. However, supplementing with natural Herbal extracts especially SASA (Japanese bamboo) extracts is very helpful. After you apply heat, the Far Infrared will remain in the body for eight hours. Therefore, do not take a bath or shower within eight hours.

First, apply heat on spine ups and down to awaken autonomic Nervous System. Then you will have some results from applying heat all over the body, but you will have a much greater impact if you find any areas yielding a strong reaction. Treat these areas, considering their relationship to the entire body. If you do not see any effect, then you are doing it incorrectly. Do not give up. Please study more or study with someone who is an expert. You can become an expert with little **ONNETSUKI** in a relatively short time. If you learn well, you can create amazing results.

For those who have very fragile skin, for example older people and very young children, you must apply a lower level of heat intensity (using the controls on **ONNETSUKI**).

This machine is very different from other heat machines because it has two or three layers of computerized safety controls. You can be at ease in using it as directed. If you use it incorrectly you could burn yourself or damage the machine. So please read the directions carefully before using.

Correct Usage:

1. If you only concentrate on an area of pain or the location to be healed, you may not get good results. You must always begin with the foundational treatment, which is fundamental to all treatment plans. Then, proceed to the use techniques described in this book for particular diseases. (pg. 70-1)

2. Use only on dry skin. Wipe cream, oil, sweat and water off.

3. Prepare **ONNETSUKI** by putting the provided cotton-cloth cap in place. Then place the cotton cloth on the patient's skin. Move the machine very smoothly and slowly in circular motions, about 10 centimeters in diameter. Gradually move toward the center and stop for one-two seconds. If it feels too hot, remove the machine from the skin or begin circular motions again.

4. A first-time user should start with low heat. Do not keep **ONNETSUKI** in one spot. Just keep moving. Once you get used to it, you can stop in the area where healing is needed.

5. The treatment usually takes 30 minutes to 1 hour.

6. If you carefully and patiently apply the heat, the areas will become pink in color and the body will feel comfortably warm and light. If the patient feels a bit sleepy, consider the heat treatment a success. Then you can stop and the patient will sleep very well that night.

7. This machine operates at 100 volts. You must use an adapter in countries that have higher voltage.

8. Please do not touch **ONNETSUKI** with wet hands, or pour water (liquid in general) on the machine.

9. The heater functions perfectly, but please don't leave it on top of paper. There s no danger of fire, because it automatically shuts off, but it can damage **ONNETSUKI**.

10. Avoid using **ONNETSUKI** on areas of inflammation and/or infection.

11. Please be careful not to burn anyone. Make sure that you always use the cotton cloth cap or sheets or cotton towel.

12. If you happen to burn someone, use Vitamin E oil, a dry, protective bandage. Such burns are caused by carelessness of the healer. There is no way you will burn somebody if you are careful.

13. Take plenty of fluid after the treatment. Also take rest after the treatment, as your energy will be used a lot when you start to heal yourself.

THE FOUNDATIONAL THERAPY

The basic maintenance and healing technique is called FOUNDATION HEALING. It must be done as the first step in any treatment plan. The Autonomic Nervous System exists alongside the spine. If you put heat along this nervous system (beginning with the nape of the neck and extending down the entire spinal column), the patient becomes very energized, no matter where the illness is. The power starts to awaken in the body and it will be easier to locate areas that need treatment once you finish this foundational healing.

Go through the entire
body, especially along
the spine, recognize
hot spots and treat.

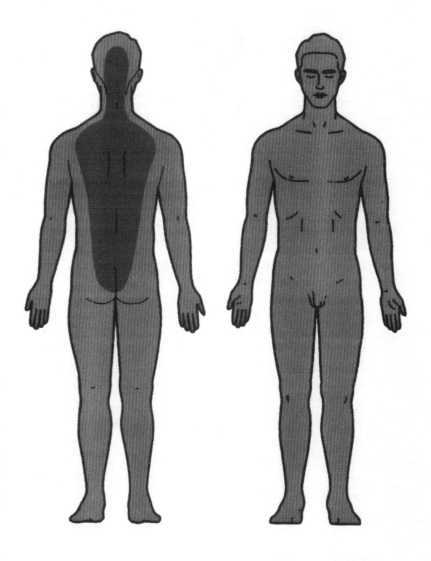

FOUNDATION HEALING A   **FOUNDATION HEALING B**

DURING AND AFTER THE TREATMENT

1. Some people have very fragile skin and will burn, even on lower heat, if you leave **ONNETSUKI** in one area too long.

2. People taking medicine especially adrenal hormone will burn more easily. You must be careful and ask about medication being taken.

3. Some people will feel very light and good while others will become very tired. Some get a little feverish, especially those who have taken a lot of medicine. Until these medicines (toxins) leave the body, the fever will persist and they may experience exhaustion and pain. These are all good reactions. Please ask patients to reduce medicines even if little by little.

4. Some people immediately take medicine for a fever. A fever is your friend. Please bear with it and do not artificially reduce your temperature. Lowering the body temperature while undergoing this therapy may result in a very high temperature. Not to worry, though, this is a good and expected reaction. You must wait and have the patient rest quietly. The fever will go down and the patient will feel very well. That's because the toxins from the medicine leave the body. For eight hours, this heat will stay in the body, so please do not take a bath.

5. With respect to food, sometimes people advise fasting. This is nonsense. You must have a balanced diet to maintain healthy cells. It is always better to eat very nutritious food and lift your own healing power than fast to kill the cancer cells. Focus mentally on the fact that you're going to build up the power of good cells and the good cells will take care of the cancer cells.

VARIOUS CANCER TREATMENTS

1. Brian Cancer

Symptoms:

Intense headache.

Intense dizziness, as if you are going to fall.

Gradual loss of sight.

Nausea and vomiting.

Sudden loss of consciousness fainting with or without seizure.

Numbness in one half of the body.

Difficulty in speech.

Difficulty in muscle movement.

Abnormal hormone production (pituitary tumors).

A feeling of having something stuck in your ear.

Sleepiness. You have no fighting spirit.

Healing Method:

Start with the foundational healing treatment to the Autonomic Nervous System, along the spine. (From now on, every treatment requires this, so I will not continue to repeat it.)

Go over all areas of the head and face. Apply heat to any area with a strong reaction. Often the back of the neck and head will react.

If there is a reaction between the eyebrows, you must make sure to apply heat here to treat the pituitary.

If there is difficulty with speech, there should be a reaction on the left side of the brain. Apply heat until this reaction subsides.

After only a few treatments, the more frequent the better, this reaction will gradually diminish.

Advise against surgery. This type of healing is very effective with brain tumors. One can heal the brain without cutting or damaging it at all. Also, you can search for the location of the cancer without cutting into the brain.

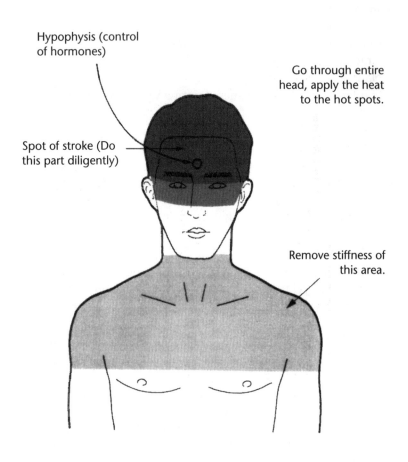

Hypophysis (control of hormones)

Go through entire head, apply the heat to the hot spots.

Spot of stroke (Do this part diligently)

Remove stiffness of this area.

BRAIN TUMOR A

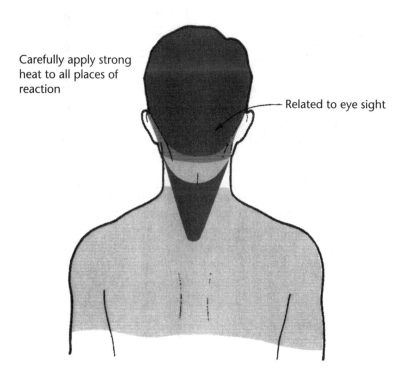

Carefully apply strong heat to all places of reaction

Related to eye sight

BRAIN TUMOR B

2. Maxillary Cancer (cancer of the upper jaw)

Symptoms:

There is always a stuffy nose with yellow or bloody mucus.

The face becomes swollen.

The inside of the mouth and upper jaw are swollen. If the patient touches it with the tongue, she does not feel pain, but does feel swelling.

Healing Method:

Use heat on the entire face; concentrate on areas of swelling.

Even if there is a reaction on only one side of the face, apply heat to both sides until the reaction subsides.

Usually it will take only one week before the reaction subsides.

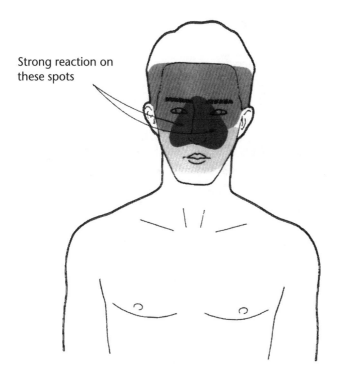

Strong reaction on
these spots

MAXILLA CANCER

3. Cancer of the Throat

Symptoms:

The voice becomes hoarse.

There is some itchiness of the throat. The patient keeps trying to clear the throat through coughing.

There is a feeling that something is stuck between the nose and eyes.

The patient coughs up mucus mixed with blood.

Healing Method:

Apply heat to the entire throat, front and back. Especially apply heat to the front under the chin.

One must also focus on the nape of the neck and back of the head.

If you notice any mold starting to grow, burn it out. Moxa may also be used.

Ear, Jaw, Throat, Chest, Nose should be carefully examined. If you find black spots, burn it out with onnetsuki.

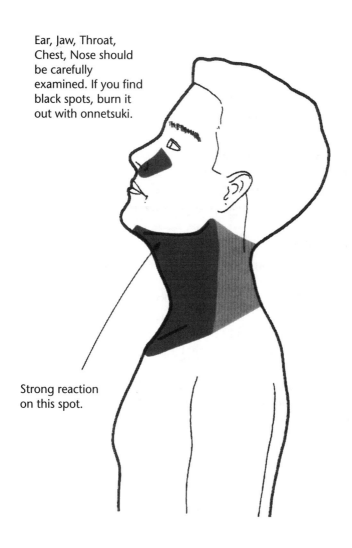

Strong reaction on this spot.

LARYNX & PHARYNX CANCER
(Throat cancer)

4. Thyroid Cancer

Symptoms:
The voice becomes hoarse.
The throat is itchy all the time.
The patient constantly tries to clear the throat.
Rapid heartbeat. Breathlessness. Dizziness.

Healing Method:
Apply heat to the entire throat (front and back) and to the back of the ear.
You should burn off any black spots.
If there is lymph node enlargement, please apply heat to the area. Very carefully apply heat to the back of the head.
Also apply heat to the adrenal and kidney areas.
Precautions:
If the patient experiences palpitations or rapid heart beat, they may see a cardiologist. This may not help them. Treating the heart won't cure them.

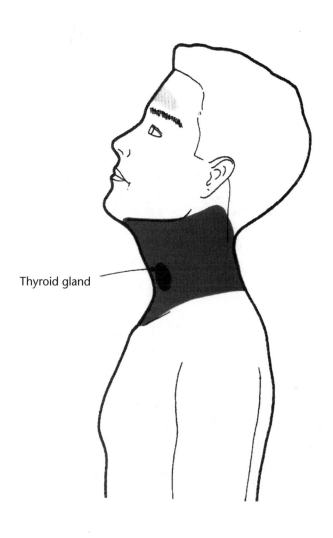

Thyroid gland

THYROID CANCER

5. Cancer of the Esophagus

Symptoms:
> The feeling that anything eaten gets stuck in the throat.
> The feeling that something is lodged in the throat.
> Heartburn. (Esophageal cancer is often misdiagnosed as stomach problems.)
> Food does not go down smoothly.
> Undigested food is vomited.
> In the last stage, one cannot even keep water down.

Healing Method:
You must treat the entire esophagus, from the top of the throat to the stomach. Then check for the exact location of the tumor.

Most of the time, it is right above the stomach or at the very beginning of the esophagus. Of course, you do the heat treatment wherever you find a strong reaction.

Gradually, the reaction lessens. Continue to treat until it is gone. Gradually, esophageal function will return, heartburn will diminish and symptoms will disappear. Esophageal cancer is easy to treat. If the patient has surgery, their life span will most definitely shorten. **ONNETSUKI** is especially effective for esophageal cancer, so please try it before surgery.

Insert heat on this area also. Strong reaction on entire esophagus area but especially these areas are most affected. upper stomach area is also affected.

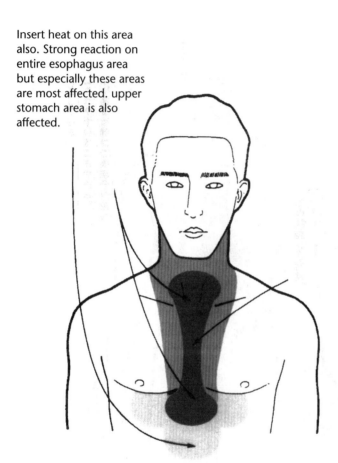

ESOPHAGEAL CANCER A

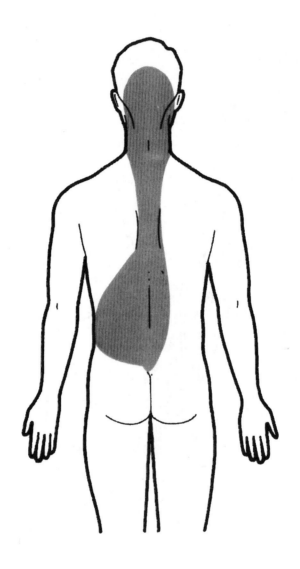

ESOPHAGEAL CANCER B

6. Stomach cancer

Stomach cancer is more common than cancer of the esophagus. The stomach is more easily affected by psychological stress. In our contemporary, modern life, sooner or later, no matter who you are, it is difficult to avoid aggravation.

Symptoms:
There are no symptoms until the cancer is quite advanced.
In the beginning, there is no pain in the stomach, but the stomach may feel very heavy.
There is a feeling of pressure that accompanies hunger.
Loss of appetite.
Nausea, if the upper part of the stomach and pylorus are affected.
Anemia and weight loss.
Pale, ashen skin color.
A mass may be felt when the stomach is touched.
The patient may spit up blood, therefore it may be misdiagnosed as an ulcer.

Healing Method:
You must apply heat, of course, to the stomach and try to find the exact location of the tumor.
Most of the time, the entire stomach is involved, so you should treat the entire stomach.
Treat the stomach area, both back and front.
Usually, cancer will also affect the duodenum, liver, and/or lung.
All other organs should be examined for a strong reaction. Try to treat them right away.

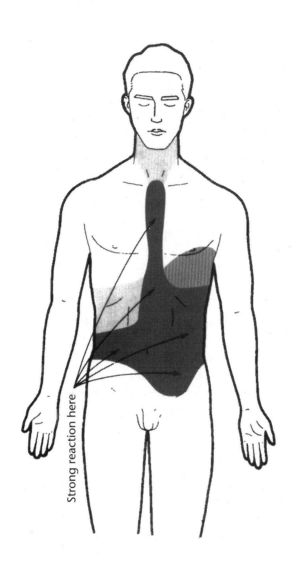

Strong reaction here

STOMACH CANCER A

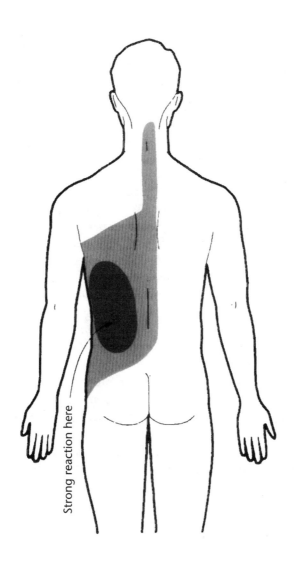

Strong reaction here

<u>STOMACH CANCER B</u>

7. Lung Cancer

Symptoms:

There are no symptoms initially.

Most lung cancers are said to be caused by cigarette smoking. I personally believe that this is not the biggest factor. It is caused more by stiffness of the shoulder and arm carrying prolonged stresses. You overwork the arm and have bad circulation there. This extends to the back. If you have poor circulation in both arms, your blood is not clear. Often this shows up first as upper arm pain.

Often, when ambient temperature changes drastically, the patient will cough very strongly and deeply.

The patient may cough up bloody sputum.

There may be pain in the scapular region of the back.

There is nerve pain in the arm. Please, when you note arm pain, always check the patient's lung area. It interested me to note that recently in Japan, we have more difficulty with lung cancer than stomach cancer. I think it is because people are overworked and using computers and machines. This leads to more back and shoulder stiffness. On the computer, you must read all these words and shapes that are not steady. The effort needed to read these shaking words creates tremendous stress. Humans are really being controlled by technology and stress is being caused by this technology. The environment is in bad condition on top of that. This type of stress causes lung cancer.

Healing Method:

Do shiatsu, especially on the upper arms and scapular region of the back. When these areas are stiff, it causes problems with circulation of the blood in the lung.

Apply heat, especially to the back.

Examine for a reaction in the frontal chest area.

Identify any areas of stabbing pain. Treat these areas. If lung cancer is advanced, it will not heal easily. Do not give up.

Carefully check the chest, arm muscles and shoulder bones.

If symptoms last a long time and coughing does not stop, pay attention more to front.

If breast cancer is present, lung cancer may be next. They often develop together.

The entire lung may be affected. Repair it if you can since you can not remove both lungs. This method can repair it.

These areas have strong
reactions (top of left lung,
bottom of right lung). Both
sides of collar bones have
also strong reactions.

Treat under the
collar bone for
severe coughing.

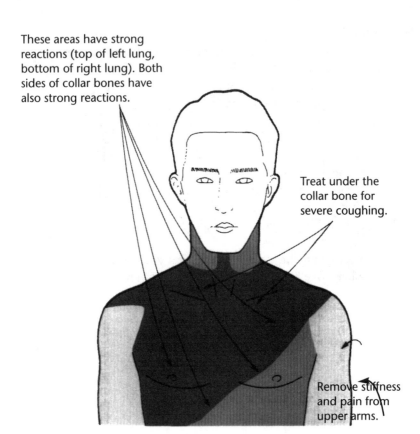

Remove stiffness
and pain from
upper arms.

LUNG CANCER A

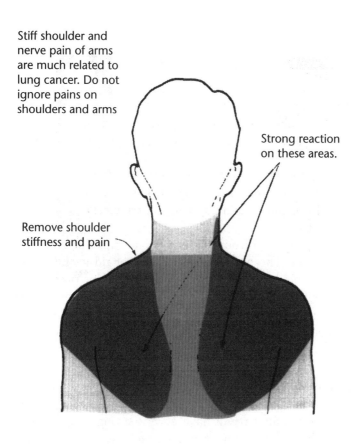

Stiff shoulder and nerve pain of arms are much related to lung cancer. Do not ignore pains on shoulders and arms

Strong reaction on these areas.

Remove shoulder stiffness and pain

LUNG CANCER B

8. Duodenal Cancer

Symptoms:

With hunger, the right side of the abdomen hurts. Often this is mistaken for stomach pain, but it is duodenal pain.

Nausea and vomiting, if the cancer is just beyond the pylorus.

Often, the entire duodenum is involved, which leads to liver problems. The patient appears jaundiced.

Pancreatic juice builds up and the pancreas becomes very painful.

Poisons released from the liver cannot travel into the duodenum. The body, therefore, cannot rid itself of toxins and they remain in the bloodstream. This often reveals itself in the skin as allergic reactions or itchiness. The breath also smells very badly. Usually, nine out of ten people have a strong reaction on this area, because the duodenum is easily affected by stress.

Healing Method:

Feel around the navel and to the right of navel. Apply heat to this area. It will have a very strong reaction: sharp stabbing like a knife. From the back, also apply heat from the fifth to the twelfth thoracic vertebrae.

You also must apply heat to the liver and spleen.

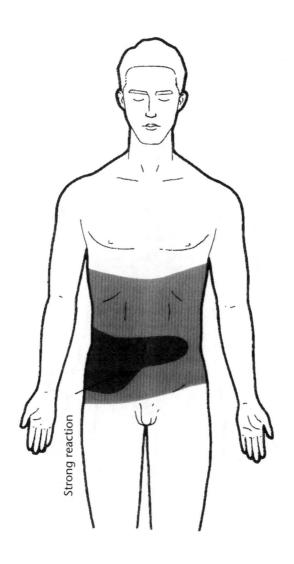

Strong reaction

DUODENAL CANCER A

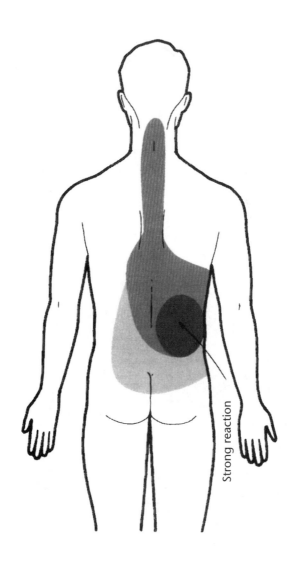

Strong reaction

DUODENAL CANCER B

9. Liver Cancer

Symptoms:
There may be no symptoms initially.
As it progresses, touching the areas may yield dull pain and
hardness. The patient may have symptoms of hepatitis.
The abdominal area expands due to water retention.

Healing Method:
Treat the liver. It is under the rib cage on the right side.
Treat the shoulder blade area on the back, especially the right side.
You must also treat the duodenum. If the duodenum in not function-
ing well, the liver will not be able to secrete properly.
Check the stomach and pancreas. All of the organs near the liver
should be treated.

10. Liver Problems (Hepatopathies)

Recently, liver problems have increased, and there has been frequent liver transplantation as a result. It is better to try to repair
your own. I think it is possible to heal yourself. It is better to treat
the duodenum rather than the liver itself.

Almost all people who have problems with their liver have
problems with their duodenum and their entire intestines are inflamed. If you have duodenal problems, all waste that the liver at-
tempts to expel remains in the liver. Later on, this gets absorbed
into the blood and induces skin problems like allergic reactions,
rashes, etc. I have recently come to believe, very strongly, that the
duodenum is the cause of many liver problems. If you apply heat
to the duodenum, very often the liver problem (like hepatitis) goes

away very quickly. The function of the duodenum is not well known and no one is paying to much attention to it.

So if the have good liver regeneration, you do not need transplantation. Pneumonia, Hepatitis A, B, C etc. all, can be helped by fixing the spleen and the duodenum. They can be healed quickly. It is very helpful to keep the kidneys clean with proper elimination. Treating the duodenum yields unbelievable results because everyone is paying attention ONLY to the liver when treating liver damage. Also remember that the liver eliminates toxins. It is important not to overwork the liver by taking too much medicine. This can harm the liver.

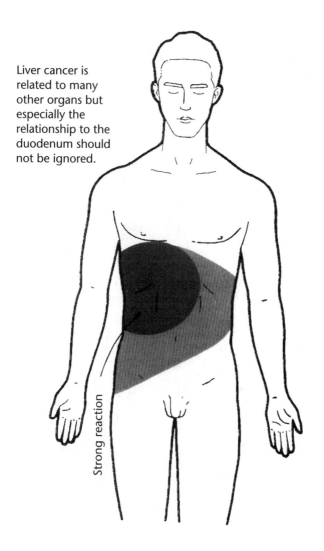

Liver cancer is related to many other organs but especially the relationship to the duodenum should not be ignored.

Strong reaction

LIVER CANCER A

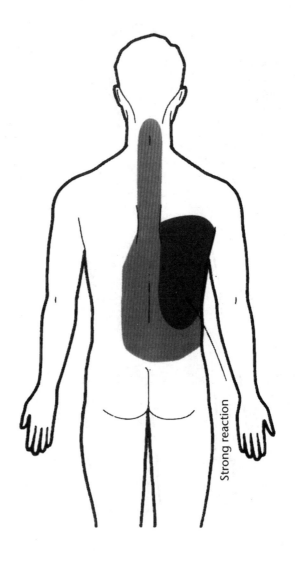

Strong reaction

LIVER CANCER B

11. Pancreatic Cancer

Symptoms:

Asymptomatic, initially.

Chronic left back pain.

Simple stomach pain.

Lower back pain that may be mistaken for nerve pain.

Pancreatic juice cannot be released leading to intense pain. It may digest the pancreas and leak out into the abdominal cavity. This is very dangerous and may lead to death.

Healing Method:

The pancreas, which opens up into the duodenum via a duct, is swollen. So, you must first heal the duodenum to restore flow.

Apply heat from the back, left side, through the front to the diaphragm area.

The relationship to other organs is very important, so you must treat all nearby organs, especially the adrenal area.

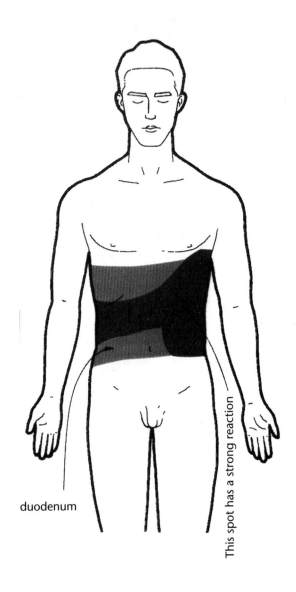

duodenum

This spot has a strong reaction

PANCREATIC CANCER A

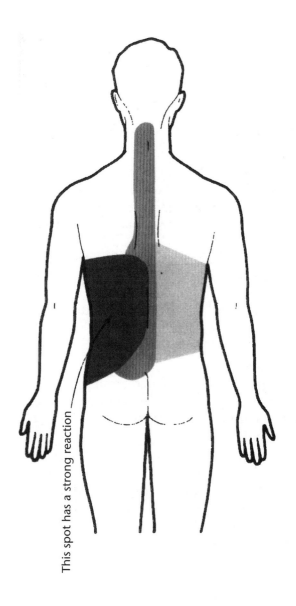

This spot has a strong reaction

PANCREATIC CANCER B

12. Bladder, Prostate and Penile Cancer

Symptoms:

One cannot sleep due to frequent urination, sometimes every half-hour through the night.

Blood in the urine, which disappears and returns. Gradually the amount of blood increases and there is a risk of hemorrhage.

Very often there is discomfort in the prostate and pressure in the rectum, perineum and anus. Urination becomes very difficult and may cease.

Residual urine is left in the bladder after urination.

The above is also applicable to penile cancer.

Healing Method:

Treat the right inguinal region in cases of bladder cancer.

You must treat the pelvis, testicles, penis, perineum, rectum, anus and inner thighs. Very often the cancer is not only in one spot.

Precautions:

This is a large, delicate, deeply rooted area. Surgery is very complex and the cancer is likely to recur. It will improve with **ONNETSUKI**. You may have a strong, very painful reaction, but it will disappear rapidly. Also, there are no side effects. People think this area is shameful and dirty, making them delay seeking treatment. It is important to seek treatment early.

Bladder cancer occurs in both men and women, more often in the older population. The lymph nodes in the groin may enlarge if they are involved. This type of cancer is very easy to treat with this heat method.

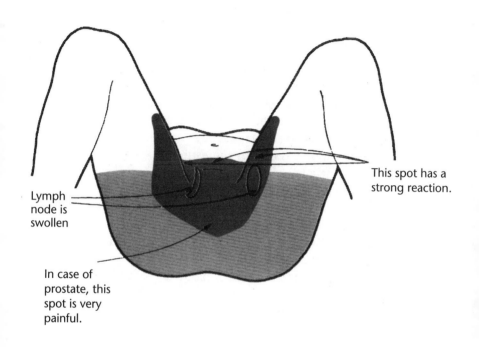

Lymph
node is
swollen

This spot has a
strong reaction.

In case of
prostate, this
spot is very
painful.

BLADDER, PROSTATE & CANCER OF THE PENIS

13. Cancer of the Large Intestine

Symptoms:

Constipation and diarrhea. (Do not take pills right away.)

Symptoms similar to those of hemorrhoids. Cancer can be mistaken for hemorrhoids.

Bloody stools—sometimes very bright red in color.

A bloated feeling in the stomach, no matter what is eaten. Since the feeling relates to the stomach, one doesn't realize the source is the large intestine.

After having a bowel movement, you don't feel completely finished.

Difficulty in having a bowel movement. It may be thin with a yellowish discharge.

There is sometimes pain in the lower abdominal area, or it feels very tense and tight.

Sometimes, a large amount of blood is passed into the toilet.

The inner thigh lymph nodes enlarge.

Healing Method:

Treat the lower abdomen and the left inner thigh.

Treat the inguinal area, where the intestine turns, as well as the duodenum.

Treat the back: thoracic area, lumbar area, tailbone, buttocks and anus.

Apply heat to all the digestive organs. This will help the bleeding gradually stop.

When the reaction to the heat treatment diminishes the bleeding stops and normal stools return the patient is getting well.

Precautions:

A patient came to me complaining of pain in the legs. I began treating for nerve pain, but when the pain didn't subside, I checked the inner thigh lymph nodes. They were swollen, so I thought of large intestinal cancer and treated it as such. Gradually, the pain went away. If I had not noticed the swollen lymph nodes, it would have been too late to treat. You cannot focus on one part of the body. You must use the entire body to diagnose.

Recently, I have seen many cases of cancer of the large intestines. People use a lot of antibiotics, which weaken your own good intestinal germs. Also, there are many chemicals in processed food, which threaten the good germs in our intestines.

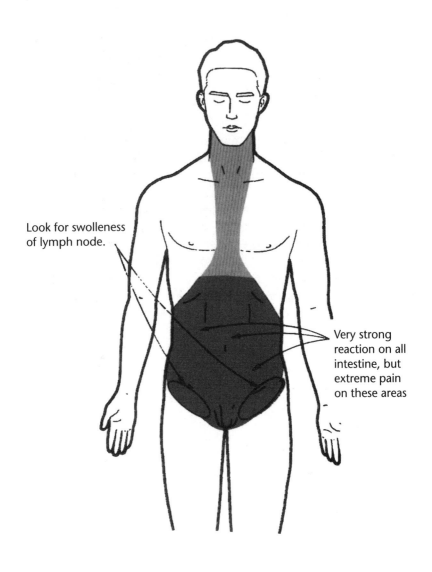

Look for swolleness
of lymph node.

Very strong
reaction on all
intestine, but
extreme pain
on these areas

CANCER OF THE LARGE INTESTINE A

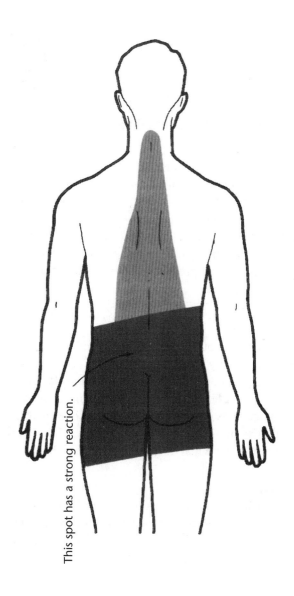

This spot has a strong reaction.

CANCER OF THE LARGE INTESTINE B

14. Cancer of the Uterus and Ovaries

Symptoms:

No obvious symptoms initially.

Bloody and smelly vaginal discharge.

Bloody, smelly vaginal discharge, which becomes constant as cancer progresses.

Hardening of the labia majora. The lymph nodes in the area become enlarged. Advise against surgery.

The more the cancer progresses, the worse smelling the yellowish discharge.

Healing Method:

Apply heat to the pubic bone, inner thigh and perineum.

Apply heat directly to the perineum and vaginal area.

You must dig in deeply to find the lymph nodes of the inner thigh. This will be a very hot, painful spot.

The reaction will subside after four or five treatments.

Also treat the pubic bone in ovarian cancer. Treat both sides, even if the reaction is only on one side.

Precautions:

When the lymph nodes of the inner thigh (inguinal area) are enlarged, you must consider the possibility of many cancers in the lower abdominal region. These include cancers of uterine, bladder, rectum, etc. With gynecological cancer, you must also treat the thyroid.

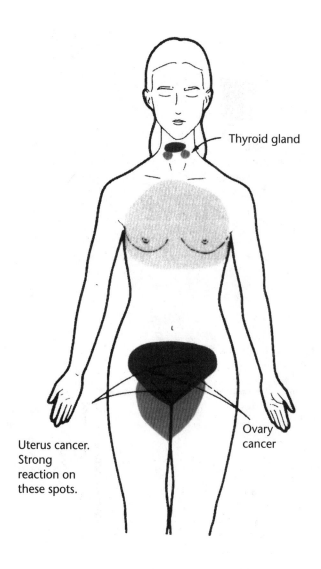

Thyroid gland

Uterus cancer.
Strong
reaction on
these spots.

Ovary
cancer

CANCER OF THE UTERUS AND OVARIES A

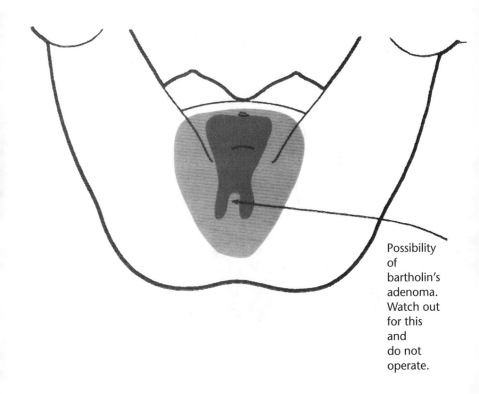

Possibility
of
bartholin's
adenoma.
Watch out
for this
and
do not
operate.

CANCER OF THE UTERUS AND OVARIES B

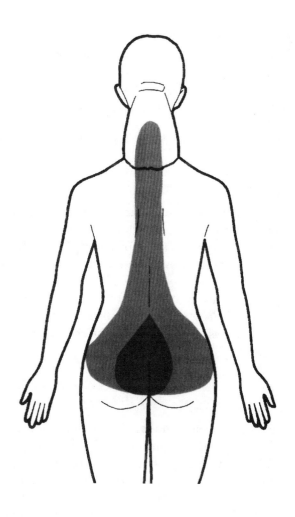

CANCER OF THE UTERUS AND OVARIES C

15. Cancer of the Breast

Symptoms:

Early on, it is very difficult to find and diagnose. It would be great if, at this stage, you could find it with **ONNET-SUKI**. It is possible to cure at this stage.

The breast is hard (mass) to the touch. It may be mistaken for a mastopathy. There may also be hardness under the armpit.

If the patient carefully checks the bosom, there maybe black spots.

Healing Method:

The patient will react with very sharp pain in the area of the breast cancer, even before it is seen on mammogram.

Check the armpit area for sharp pain with **ONNETSUKI.**

Carefully apply heat all over the breast area. The pain will go away rapidly.

If there are any black spots or blackening of the skin, burn them off with **ONNETSUKI.** Advise against surgery.

To see if the disease has spread deeply, check for a reaction on the back, arms, and abdominal area.

16. Other Cancers

Skin cancer, bone cancer, lymphoma, eye cancer, muscle cancer—cancer appears anywhere. Using **ONNETSUKI**, one should be able to find the sharp pain spot at any part of the body, and treat it and diagnose cancer before it shows up on X-rays. Diligently and patiently apply heat to these areas and the pain will usually subside. **ONNETSUKI** can be used in areas where surgery is impossible. Skin cancer or muscle cancer takes a little longer to treat. Cancer of the inner organs is treated more rapidly. Cancer is not that scary.

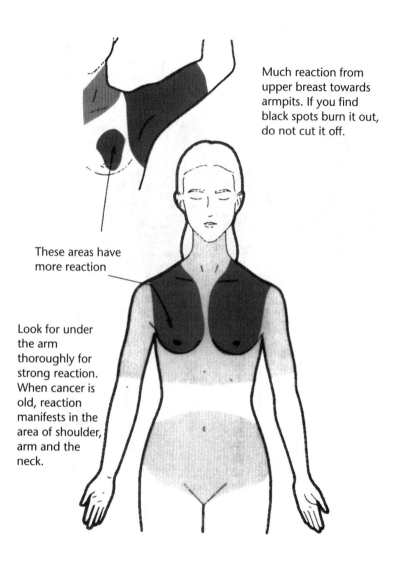

Much reaction from upper breast towards armpits. If you find black spots burn it out, do not cut it off.

These areas have more reaction

Look for under the arm thoroughly for strong reaction. When cancer is old, reaction manifests in the area of shoulder, arm and the neck.

CANCER OF THE BREAST A

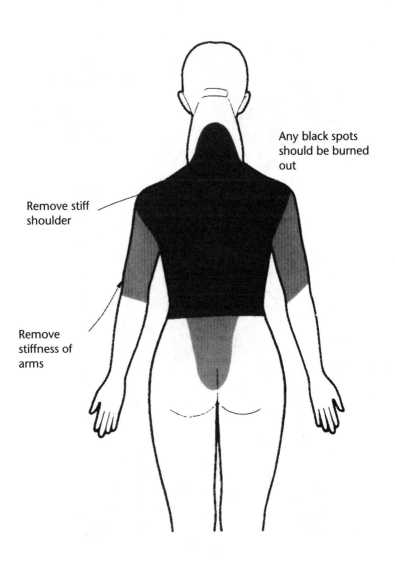

Any black spots should be burned out

Remove stiff shoulder

Remove stiffness of arms

CANCER OF THE BREAST B

Chapter 5

Treatment of Other Difficult Diseases

SOME DISEASES CANNOT BE DETECTED by technology today, possibly because they are functional illnesses. You may not be able to find any cause using Western methods and without knowing the cause, the cure cannot be found. These diseases are called nambyo in Japan. They include Parkinson's disease, Meniere's disease, Raynaud's disease, collagen vascular disease, and many others.

These diseases improve rapidly with this heat treatment. They are difficult if you try to treat them with any medicines, but they are not so difficult if you encourage the patients' own healing power. Again and again, I say nothing is unnecessary in the body. We can always find the cause of an illness. Disease is caused when some area of the body becomes unbalanced, leading to deterioration. Take, for example, chronic fatigue syndrome. In my experience, this condition often stems from a hormonal imbalance often associated with the thyroid gland. The surface skin above the gland reacts strongly to **ONNETSUKI**.

The following is a list of other illnesses related to thyroid problems: Rheumatoid arthritis, asthma, Parkinson's disease, diabetes, Meniere's disease, Autonomic Nervous System dysfunction, kidney failure, psychological disturbances, depression, insomnia, Dwarfism, infertility, menopause, low blood pressure, etc. These disorders arise in some region of the body in addition to the thyroid gland. Surgery is not wise. The function of the thyroid gland is not limited to the production of thyroid hormone.

Neurological disease is difficult to treat conventionally, but with **ONNETSUKI** the problem can be pinpointed and treated with eye-opening results. Nerve pain appears all over the body because it is traveling through the nervous system. Common problem areas include the rib cage, hip joints and face. Doctors give an injection to stop the pain. This blocks healing, so when the nerve becomes active again, the pain resumes. **ONNETSUKI** is very effective on such pain.

Lower back pain has three causes typically: 1) internal spine pain, 2) back and spinal muscle spasms, and 3) stiffness of frontal abdominal muscles. Often doctors say there is a slipped disc or that the spinal column is deformed and distorted and recommend surgery. It is very dangerous to operate on the spine. It is the main pillar of the body. If you avoid surgery and use this heat method, you may avoid living the rest of your life in a wheelchair. Lower back pain can be very painful, but if one can walk, even with great pain, it implies that the spine is healthy. Therefore, it is likely that muscles are affected. You should first carefully treat the abdominal muscles and muscles around the spine.

Doctors often say that knee pain arises when the cartilage covering bone in the joint space is worn away and damaged. I believe that most of the time the pain is caused by the nerve that innervated the knee area. The pain will go away with treatments along the tender spots found along the spine when **ONNETSUKI** is applied from the nape of the neck to the tailbone. Sports injuries such as tennis elbow are also similar and respond well to this treatment plan. "Fifty-year-old shoulder" occurs when the arm is damaged by overuse. It is important to remember that lung cancer will produce the same quality of pain in the arm.

This heat system is good for allergies, insect bites and babies' vomiting reaction to breast milk.

DIABETES

Diabetes is a disease that is without cure for a long time. Doctors and nutritionists advise diet control and weight loss. Modern medicine does not know how one becomes diabetic or how to cure it. They say that even if you eat a little, you have "sugar." If you eat more, you have more "sugar." Therefore, patients are instructed to reduce the amount of food intake. I think this approach is incorrect. Sugar levels go up and down independent of the amount of food intake. If you carefully observe, you soon learn that sugar levels have nothing to do with how much you eat. Therefore, this starvation diet approach is nonsense. Some people inherit abnormalities of the pancreas causing dysfunction. For these people, the disease is impossible to cure. For others, it is not impossible to cure. I believe this disease comes from psychological and physical stress caused by one's environment and Autonomic Nervous System imbalance caused by abnormal hormonal discharge. Non-insulin dependent diabetes is also caused by the abnormal discharge of insulin in the body. When the Autonomic Nervous System loses balance, there will be bad effects on the body. One will easily become sick. Diabetes and cancer are caused originally by Autonomic Nervous System imbalance, specifically, the sympathetic and parasympathetic nervous systems, which oppose one another, are not balanced. Our goal is to restore this balance. If the imbalance is chronic, the disease (diabetes or cancer) becomes incurable. One can treat diabetes very effectively with *ONNETSUKI*.

Cutting calories can have detrimental effects. Strict diets are nonsense; they don't work. When insulin injections are used for a period of time, the diabetes becomes incurable because the pancreas becomes dependent on the shots, produces fewer hormones and becomes lazy.

Some people are diabetic even though their pancreas functions effectively. This disease is related to adrenal and thyroid hormones along with an imbalance in the sympathetic and parasympathetic nervous systems. You cannot cure diabetes with injections, but you can treat it with **ONNETSUKI** by identifying hot areas and applying heat to restore balance. I have often seen patients' sugar count returns to normal after one treatment! Of course, the outcome of treatment depends on the patient. I recommend eating normally and having heat treatments daily. One patient talked about this treatment in the hospital. The doctor said it was impossible. The patient reported that he had been eating normally. The doctor thought this was crazy and asked the patient to stop the heat treatments. However, it worked! Why should it be stopped?

Over-production of adrenaline can cause obesity. Diabetes is associated with obesity, but it doesn't mean that because all obese people will get diabetes. Starving oneself is dangerous because there is a loss of important life force energy, risk of malnutrition and risk of nerve damage.

Treatment:

i) Heat back, spine, adrenal and kidney areas.

ii) Heat liver, duodenum, and pancreas (left upper abdomen) in the front.

iii) Heat the throat in the thyroid area.

iv) Heat between eyebrows—the important "order center" for hormones.

v) Depending on the patient, any number or all of these areas may react. In any case, treat each area affected until the reaction lessens.

Patients should eat well-balanced meals. It is not necessary to starve. Even with normal pancreatic function, other hormonal dysfunction may lead to insulin suppression and diabetes. Pancreatic dysfunction is not the only cause of diabetes, so remember to carefully examine all the other areas mentioned above.

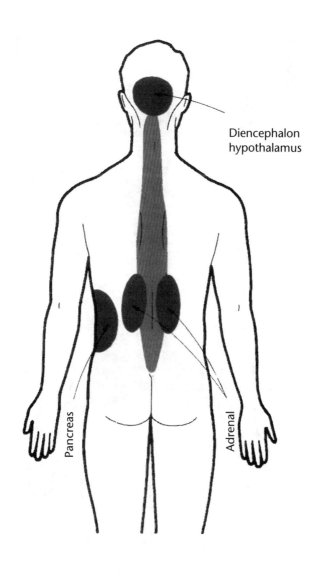

Diencephalon
hypothalamus

Pancreas

Adrenal

DIABETES A

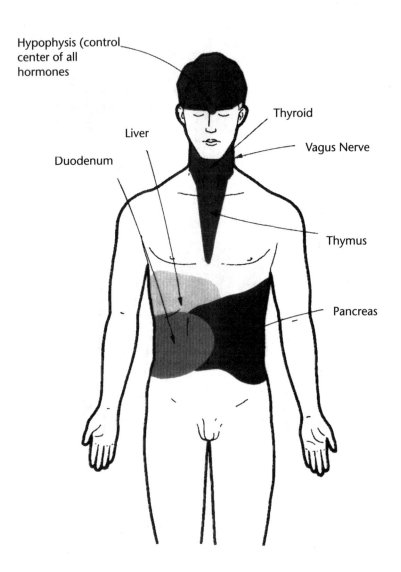

Hypophysis (control center of all hormones

Thyroid

Vagus Nerve

Liver

Duodenum

Thymus

Pancreas

DIABETES B

EYE DISEASES

1. Cataract—Poor lymphatic circulation in the eye causes the lens to become opaque. This can happen as a side effect of medicine or be caused by decreased eye muscle activity. Applying Far Infrared heat to the eyeballs is very effective. Remove contact lenses and apply heat directly to the eyeball and around the eyes.

2. Dryness of Eyes—Tears are diminished due to pain from contact lenses or rubbing the eyes. Sometimes one cannot keep the eyes open, even with eye drops.

3. Dacyostenosis—Tears run through to the nose and this channel becomes inflamed.

4. Apollo Disease—The eye becomes very red due to a viral infection. Doctors have a difficult time treating this. No fever is present. It is very contagious. It is so named because the disease flourished in the year Apollo reached the moon. The virus is very weak when exposed to heat, therefore, **ONNETSUKI** is very effective.

5. Stye—This inflammatory growth of the eyelid is caused by extreme fatigue and Vitamin A deficiency. Be careful of cutting them because they will re-emerge and can spread over the face. You can use the heat method.

6. Star Eye—A very painful growth in the eyes.

7. General Fatigue of the Eyes—Vision decreases when the eyes are tired. One may experience headaches, nausea and difficulty reading.

8. Pollinosis—A seasonal (more in spring) nasal allergic reaction. Very often it is caused by pollen from cedar and other trees. In these cases, not only the nose, but also the eyes and entire face may be affected. Other times it is caused by central heating, the nasal membranes weaken as a greenhouse flower suddenly catching a cold wind. Sensitivity to cold air can cause an allergic reaction. These cases are more common.

Heat treatment is very effective for all the conditions mentioned above (1-8).

Cataract, dacyostenosis,
xerophthalmia, tear eyes

Xerophthalmia
(dryness of the
eyeball)

Cataract—strong
reaction under the
eyes and near the
nose.

Dacyostenosis
(narrowness
of tear tube)

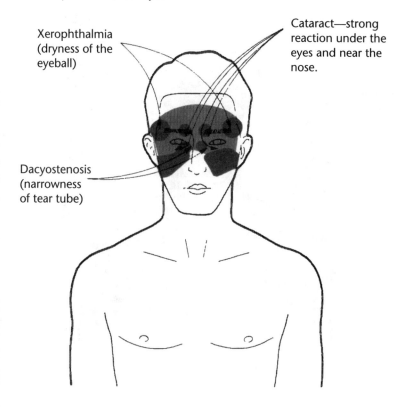

EYE A

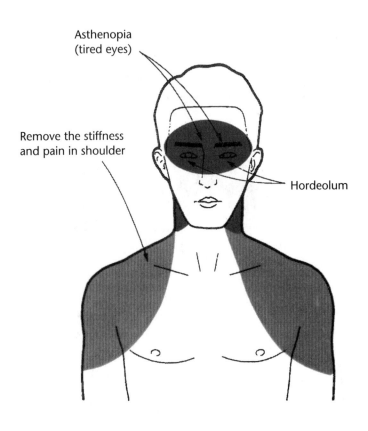

Asthenopia
(tired eyes)

Remove the stiffness
and pain in shoulder

Hordeolum

EYE B

Hordeolum, asthenopia, lack of vitamins A&B.

Strong reaction on cornea; insert heat above eyelid.

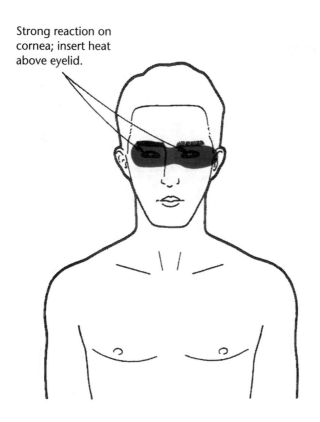

EYE C
Star eyes

Cover the area with cloth and insert heat (take off contact lenses)

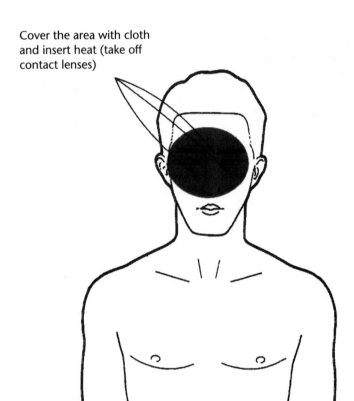

<u>EYE D</u>
Pollinosis, eye itchiness

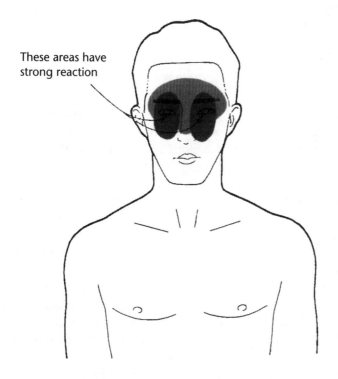

These areas have
strong reaction

<u>EYE E</u>
Apollo disease

DISEASE OF THE HEART AND ARTERIES

1. Irregular Heartbeat—You must apply heat in the thyroid and lymph node areas.

2. Thrombosis—When the vascular system becomes narrow, one will experience symptoms of numbness in the hands and legs, coldness, and pins & needles. Both small and large veins may be involved. Walking is very difficult and very painful. Gradually, the tips of your fingers and toes are affected, lose their blood supply and the tissue dies. This results in the need for finger and toe amputation. The vessels feeding the skin of the fingers and toes may be involved leading to pustulosis. The skin on the back of the legs may be involved and is not easily cured. This is one of the most difficult to cure.

The above is caused by the abnormality of the sympathetic nervous system which creates the imbalance in the veins. The application of heat in the areas often causes the symptoms to subside therefore eliminating the need for amputation. Raynaud's disease is in the same family of disease. I have been surprised and impressed over and over again by the rapid improvement of these conditions with just a few days of treatment. you can also treat the legs if they are simply tired or itchy.

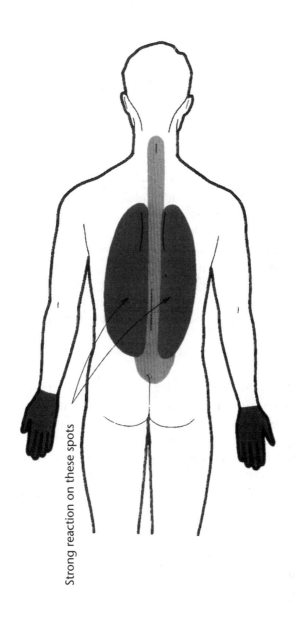

Strong reaction on these spots

CHROMBOANGIITIS OBLITERAMS, RAYNAUD'S SYNDROME

SKIN DISEASE

1. Atopic Dermatitis and Acne—They are caused by an allergy. The skin is constantly itchy or painful. There are two possible reasons for this—parasites or an underlying disorder of inner organs. If the problem is caused by parasites, creams should not be used because they may make the problem worse. Candida and Tinea are very weak fungi when exposed to heat. So **ONNETSUKI** is very effective. You may also use very hot water.

Skin problems arising from inner organ dysfunction are often linked to duodenal problems. This occurs when the ducts that eliminate toxic substances from the liver into the duodenum do not work very well. The toxins accumulate in the liver and are reabsorbed into the bloodstream. The body tries to expel them through the skin, causing itching. Most people who itch have a duodenal problem. If you treat the duodenal area, you can effectively deal with the skin disease in one or two treatments.

2. Herpes Zoster (shingles)—The chicken pox virus goes into the nervous system and sleeps before showing up on the skin in old age. It shows up on half of the body. It is so painful that if someone walks by, the air current can hurts. Loud sounds can hurts. The virus often lives inside the spine. When one is tired and weak, it recurs. People say that you get immunity and that it will not recur but I myself have had it twice.

The virus is weakened by heat. Thus, it is possible to cure it with **ONNETSUKI**. Carefully treat the spine and kill the virus so it won't recur. You can treat the affected area directly in the case of Herpes simplex. The duodenal area should be treated in most dermatological diseases. You also must treat the liver area.

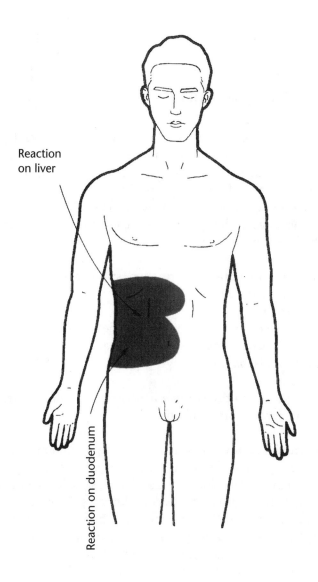

Reaction
on liver

Reaction on duodenum

SKIN DISEASE
(Skin allergy, Atopic dermatitis)

URINARY TRACT INFECTION

1. Bladder Infection—You experience urine leakage and pain during urination. The infection, caused by germs, occurs more commonly in women. You can take antibiotics, but it is not easy to cure. It recurs often for many years. The germs seem to remain dormant and reappear when the body is weak. Heat treatment is incredibly effective. If the spot where the germs are hiding can be found, the infection may be cured.

2. Anuria (no urination)—Urination stops, the body swells thereby increasing body weight. It is a difficult disease in Japan. This effects the kidneys as they experience increased back pressure from the swollen bladder and causes decreased urine formation. It may incite prostate cancer. Heat treatment to the parathyroid glands is very effective.

3. Protein spills into the urine when kidney function decreases making protein re-absorption impossible.

4. Contracted Kidney—It is a very serious condition resulting from chronic, worsening function of the kidney. Life span is quickly shortened. Kidney cells do not recycle. The cause is an abnormality in the artery that nourishes the kidney. Nutrients do not reach the kidney, therefore its function deteriorates. What causes the arterial narrowing? I think it is a sympathetic nerve disorder. The disease progresses slowly with no symptoms initially. It may be too late when symptoms begin. Treatment is focused on the sympathetic nervous system. I wonder if cardiac arrhythmia and brain tumors arise from the same sympathetic nervous system problem. Perhaps it is related to thyroid dysfunction or high blood pressure medication. If you undergo surgery, the kidney function drops to zero, obviously. The kidney is a very important organ. The kidney is the key to health, therefore you should not remove it, but try to promote its health. You must always thank your kidneys and take care of them. This kind of mental attitude is essential.

5. Bed-Wetting—It is normal to wet the bed in childhood. It is abnormal to bed wet in high school. Parents get angry, which is not healthy for a small child. Bed-wetting is due to illness. After about 300cc of urine accumulates in the bladder, one gets the urge to urinate. The nervous system control makes you wait. The control is working all the time. Bedwetting occurs when the nervous system does not function during sleep. No matter how angry you are with a child while he is awake, the situation will not improve. If you scold, the child becomes more and more unstable mentally. The symptoms may escalate. The nerve needs to be stimulated. Sometimes the hot spot can be found in the sympathetic chain of the spine, the ureter, and around the bladder. When you find these hot spots and apply heat quickly, it is possible to cure. Do not be shy: one should talk about such matters. If parents are very strict and hurt the child's feelings, the child becomes stressed and will wet the bed more. Quarreling between parents can affect the child in the same way.

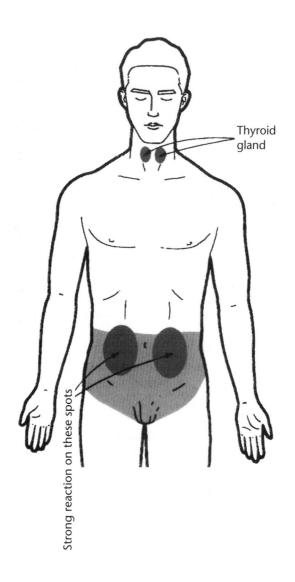

Thyroid gland

Strong reaction on these spots

URINARY TRACT DISEASES A
(anuria, proteinuria)

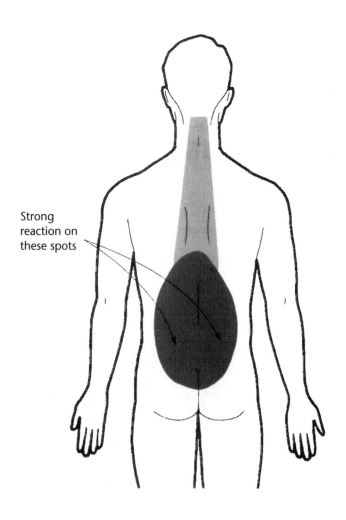

Strong
reaction on
these spots

URINARY TRACT DISEASES B
(anuria, proteinuria)

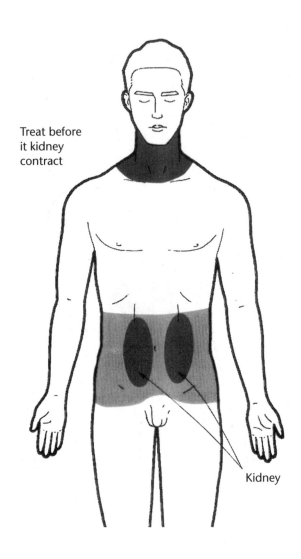

Treat before
it kidney
contract

Kidney

URINARY TRACT DISEASES C-1
(contracted kidney 1)

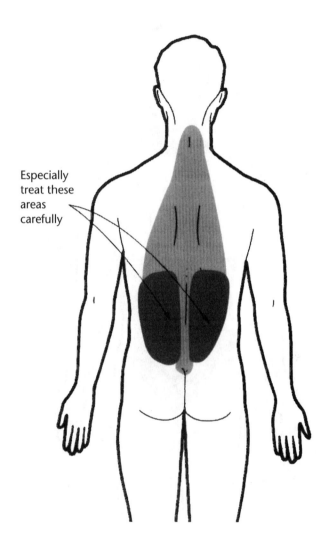

Especially
treat these
areas
carefully

URINARY TRACT DISEASES C-2
(contracted kidney 2)

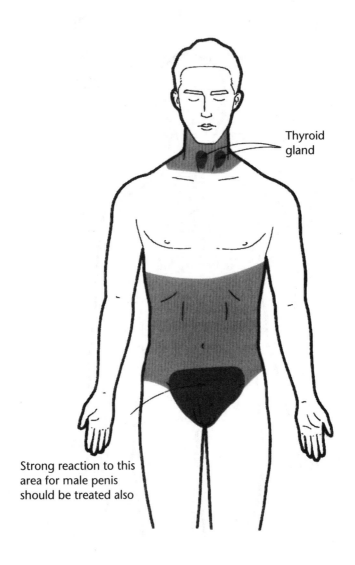

Thyroid
gland

Strong reaction to this
area for male penis
should be treated also

URINARY TRACT DISEASES D-1
(nocturnal enuresis—bed wetting 1)

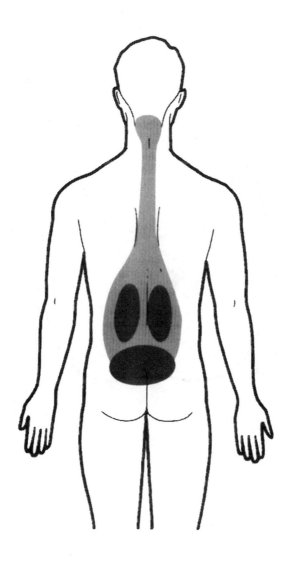

URINARY TRACT DISEASES D-2
(nocturnal enuresis—bed wetting 2)

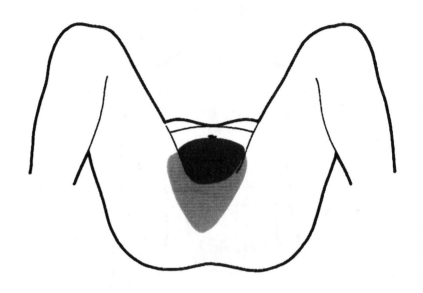

URINARY TRACT DISEASES D-3
(nocturnal enuresis—bed wetting 3)

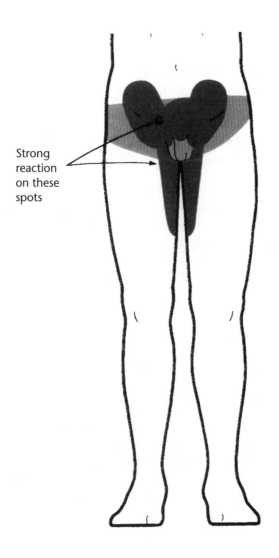

Strong
reaction
on these
spots

URINARY TRACT DISEASES E
(cystitus)

RESPIRATORY SYSTEM

1. Cough—There are many reasons for cough, so don't keep taking cough medicine. It could be bronchitis, tracheal inflammation, or an infection of the lung. It also could be lung cancer or liver enlargement. It could be caused by stiffness of the shoulder or back. For these reasons, one must first identify the cause and then plan the treatment. *ONNETSUKI* detects the location of the problem, so heat can easily be applied to the most effective area and symptoms go away naturally.

For example, a lady came taking many medications for diabetes. The medicine was damaging her liver. The liver was very swollen and pushed upon her lung. She was coughing a lot and taking cough medicine, which affected her stomach. So she took stomach medicine too. Her cough didn't stop. I asked her to stop taking the medicine for diabetes. Swelling of her liver diminished and she stopped coughing.

2. Stuffy Nose—

    a) Maxillary cancer (cancer of the upper jaw) may cause a bloody nose. It recurs after surgery.

    b) Pollen allergy may not be only caused by pollen. Heating and air-conditioning systems are the culprit. We live in such hot rooms and suddenly change when we go out into the cold air. This unnatural system causes the inner nose area to weaken. Viruses easily enter and live there. The affected person not only will suffer from the nose, but also in the eyes, cheeks and throat. The heat method is very effective with these symptoms.

    c) Inflammation and swollen nasal membranes cause stuffy nose making it difficult to breathe. A patient of mine had problems with the nose and eyes and kept going to the doctor. He didn't get well and became very depressed. I discovered a problem with the trigeminal nerve. He became well after treatments with *ONNETSUKI*.

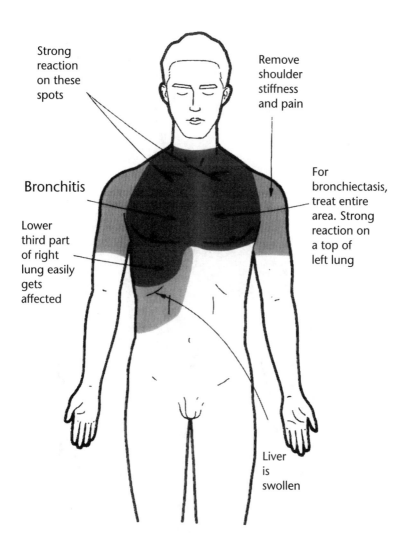

Strong reaction on these spots

Remove shoulder stiffness and pain

Bronchitis

Lower third part of right lung easily gets affected

For bronchiectasis, treat entire area. Strong reaction on a top of left lung

Liver is swollen

RESPIRATORY SYSTEM

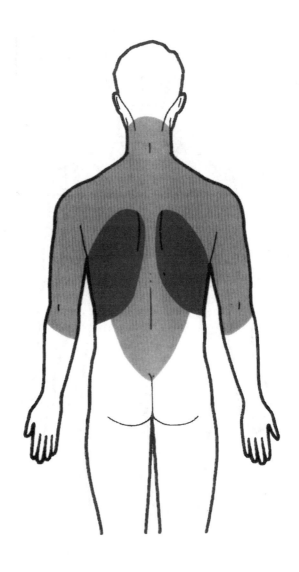

RESPIRATORY SYSTEM A
Cough 2

Strong
reaction on
these spots.
Remove
contact lenses

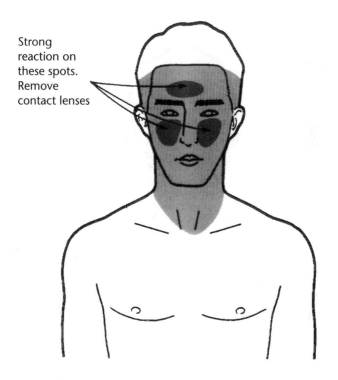

RESPIRATORY SYSTEM B
Nose 1—empyema, pollinosis, stuffed nose,
nose bleeding from maxilla cancer

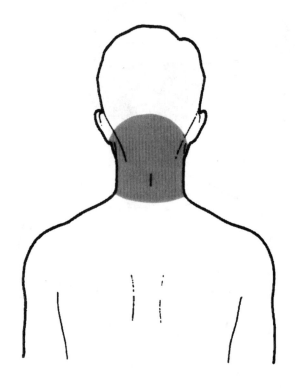

RESPIRATORY SYSTEM B
Nose 2

THE DIGESTIVE SYSTEM

Problems of the digestive organs are caused more by stress than overeating.

1. **Lack of saliva**—Saliva contains digestive enzymes, lymph fluid, detoxifiers and hormones. The saliva regulates body rhythms. Without it, the inner mouth is rough and dry. You cannot even speak very well. The rhythmic body movements become crazy. If we put heat on the salivary secretion lines, secretion will quickly be restored.

2. **Heartburn**—One experiences burning in the stomach. The upper stomach, towards the esophagus, is inflamed and this can occur with esophageal cancer.

3. **Vomiting**—Inflammation of the entrance of the stomach (cardia) or the exit of the stomach (pylorus) causes nausea. If these areas narrow or shrink, vomiting occurs. The same occurs along with inability to tolerate food with swelling of the large intestine.

4. **Gastric ulcer**—Stress and/or medicines cause this. Of course, severe cases cause the stomach wall and arteries to break down resulting in bleeding.

5. **Duodenal ulcer**—Many people do not realize that they have duodenal inflammation. Often this can present itself as liver disease. The biliary ducts may not be fully open. Very rarely is disease of the liver solely caused by a liver problem. There is almost always some kind of abnormality in the duodenum. Therefore, if a patient has any illness related to the liver, one must always check the duodenum and treat it first. If the duodenal area is healed, often the liver recovers on its own. Pancreatic juice also goes through the duodenum. If the area is clogged, juice cannot enter the duodenum smoothly. It builds up in the pancreas and may digest the pancreas. This causes tremendous abdominal pain. In this case, the duodenum should also be treated first. Do not have surgery to resect the pancreas. It is curable using the heat treatments.

The duodenum is a very important organ, which the medical world really underestimates. It is one of the most important and easily treated areas for problems in the pancreas, kidney and liver.

6. Hemorrhoids—an unpleasant nuisance. They appear with bleeding and itching in the anal area. You must not focus treatment on the anus, but on the entire digestive system. The function of the entire digestive system is weak, especially the large intestine. Even if it is operated on, it will recur. The heat method is very effective without surgery. **Fistula ani** may be caused by tubercle bacilli. The nest of the disease is very deep and can extend to the buttock. There may be copious amounts of yellow discharge. *ONNETSUKI* can help release the discharge and promote healing.

7. Tumor-like intestinal inflammation—This condition is both painful and difficult. Ulcers are present along with blood and mucus. It is caused by parasympathetic nervous system weakness. Therefore, it is easy to treat with *ONNETSUKI*. I have a 90 percent improve rate.

8. Polyps of the Large Intestine—The traditional treatment is polypectomy. However, there is no need because they very easily decrease in size with heat treatment. The benefit is that there is no intervention and harm to inner organs.

9. Diarrhea and Constipation—There are many causes of diarrhea and constipation.

a) Diarrhea can occur because something toxic was eaten and the body is working to eliminate it quickly. This type of diarrhea should never be stopped, but stimulated.

b) A weakened parasympathetic system will sometimes induce diarrhea or constipation. Medical books claim that decreased parasympathetic drive causes constipation and increased parasympathetic drive causes diarrhea. In my opinion, both can occur with weakened drive. Therefore, I give a good energy boost to the parasympathetic system in either case. If the symptoms continue for a long time, examine the patient's medication list. Some medicines that reduce stomach acid also unbalance the nervous system. Taking too many digestive pills decreases stomach function by making the parasympathetic system lazy and can result in stomach pain.

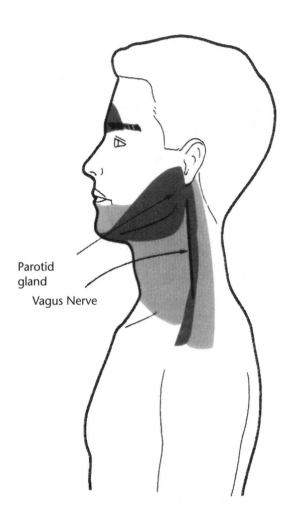

Parotid
gland

Vagus Nerve

DIGESTIVE SYSTEM A
(lack of saliva)

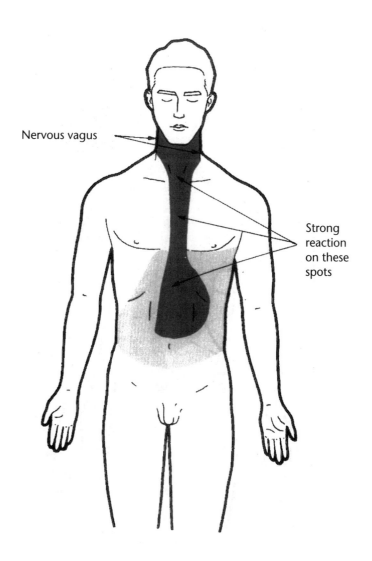

Nervous vagus

Strong
reaction
on these
spots

DIGESTIVE SYSTEM B
(heart burn 1)

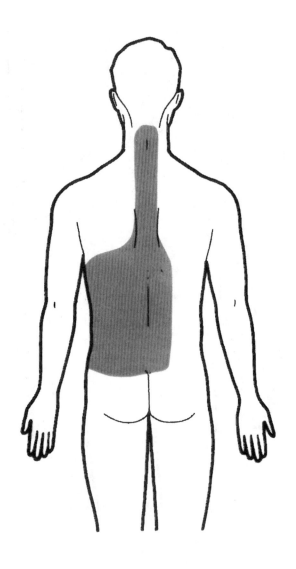

DIGESTIVE SYSTEM B
(heart burn 2)

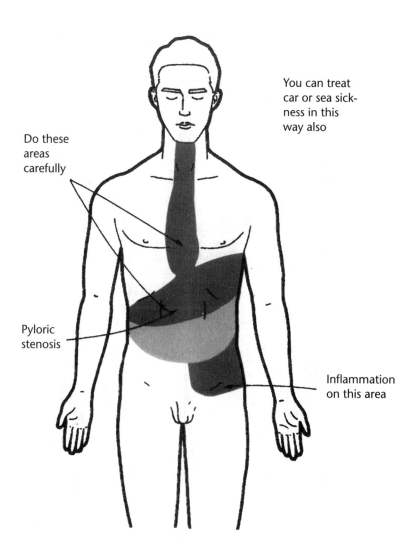

You can treat car or sea sickness in this way also

Do these areas carefully

Pyloric stenosis

Inflammation on this area

DIGESTIVE SYSTEM C
(Vomitus 1)

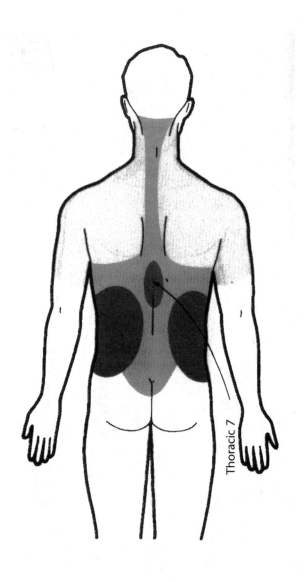

Thoracic 7

DIGESTIVE SYSTEM C
(Vomitus 2)

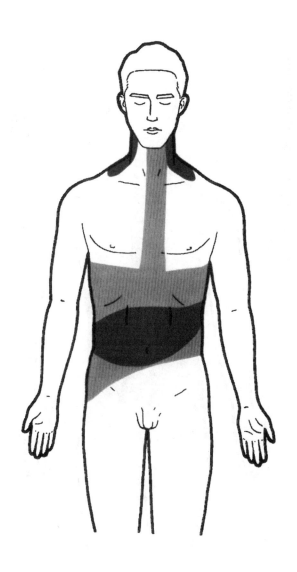

DIGESTIVE SYSTEM D
(duodenum ulcer 1)

TREATMENT OF OTHER DIFFICULT DISEASES 139

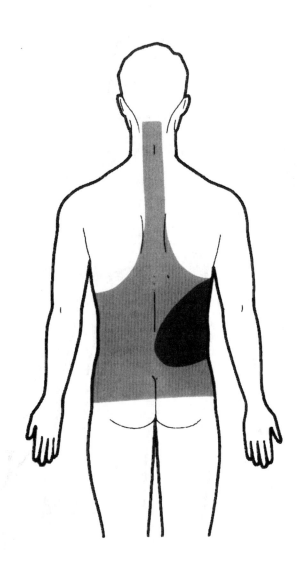

DIGESTIVE SYSTEM D
(duodenum ulcer 2)

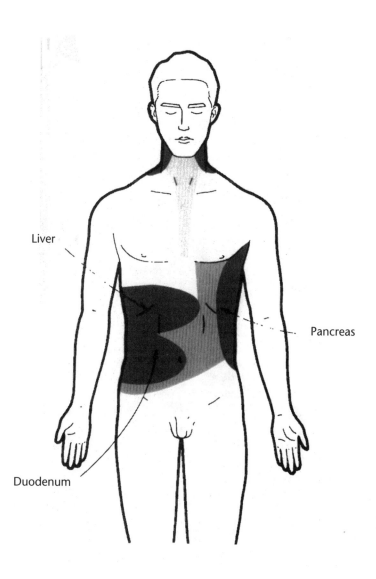

Liver

Pancreas

Duodenum

DIGESTIVE SYSTEM E
(Pancreas inflammation, Liver inflammation 1)

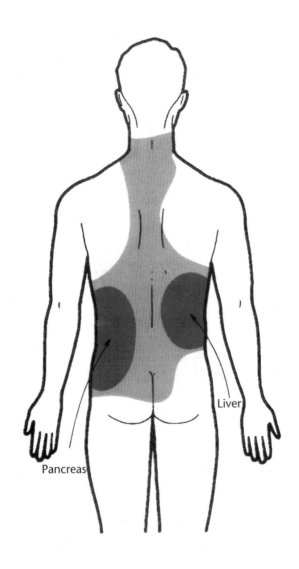

DIGESTIVE SYSTEM E
(Pancreas inflammation, Liver inflammation 2)

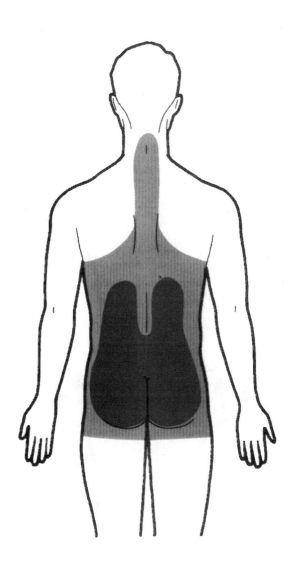

DIGESTIVE SYSTEM F
(Various hemorrhoids 1)

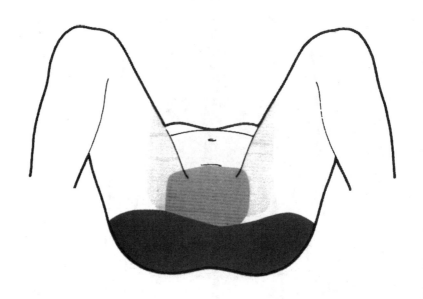

DIGESTIVE SYSTEM F
(Various hemorrhoids 2)

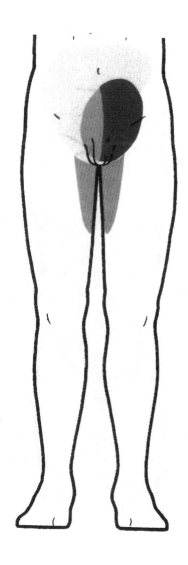

DIGESTIVE SYSTEM F
(Various hemorrhoids 3)

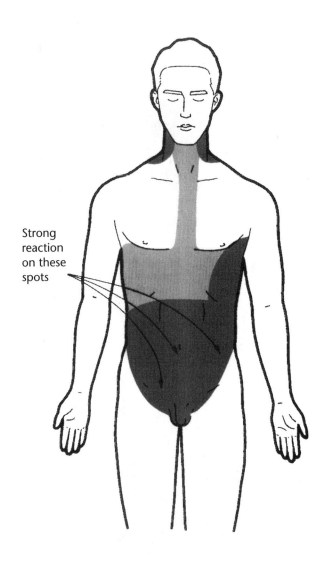

Strong reaction on these spots

DIGESTIVE SYSTEM G
(Various large intestine inflammation, polyp 1)

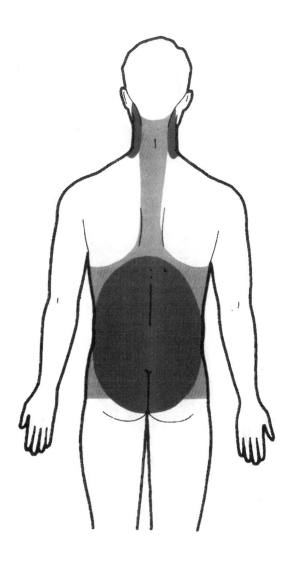

DIGESTIVE SYSTEM G
(Various large intestine inflammation, polyp 2)

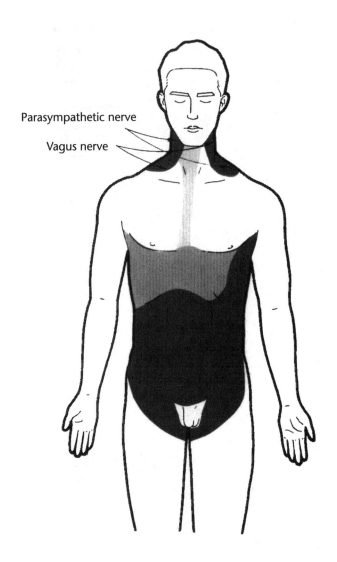

Parasympathetic nerve

Vagus nerve

DIGESTIVE SYSTEM H
(diarrhea and constipation 1)

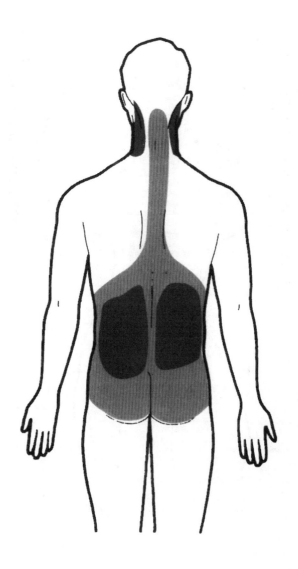

DIGESTIVE SYSTEM H
(diarrhea and constipation 2)

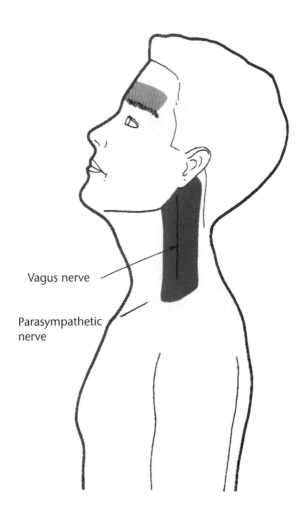

Vagus nerve

Parasympathetic nerve

DIGESTIVE SYSTEM H
(diarrhea and constipation 3)

THYROID

Thyroid-related disease include Rheumatoid arthritis, asthma, irregular heartbeat, Diabetes, Parkinson's disease, Meniere's disease, Autonomic Nervous System disorder, various kidney disease, aphasia, mental disorders, depression, insomnia, menopause, low blood pressure. There are many others, but there is a lack of studies in this area. I believe that infertility and other gynecological disease are also related.

Thyroid problems are often operated on. Stop thinking that cutting is the way to cure. It is very important that all organs are kept intact, as much as possible. I have read a medical text in which a doctor wrote that the spleen might be removed. I was shocked and angry. The spleen is such an important organ. It cannot be cut out so easily. No organs, anything in the body, are unnecessary. Every organ is related to the others. If one is lacking, many disorders will arise. Parts of cars and airplanes may be removed, but this cannot be done with the human body casually. Try to mend what you have. This is a subject of great importance.

1. Meniere's disease results in dizziness and vomiting. It is not easy to cure and causes much suffering. Medical books report a problem in the inner ear. The Japanese government classifies it as nambyo. Western medicine also considers it a difficult disease to treat. I believe this disease is caused by an imbalance of the thyroid gland. I actually have cured it by treating the thyroid. It was very simple to cure in one or two treatments. I do not understand, therefore, why it is a difficult disease.

2. Headache—It may be caused by nerve pain, trigeminal neuralgia. The thyroid may also be the cause. The pain can be very strong, so each area must be checked.

3. Depression—Mental and spiritual instability occurs when the thyroid is not functioning well. The patient may go suddenly from happy and cheerful to quiet and depressed. The patient may be placed in a psychiatric hospital if the problem is in the thyroid, but the psychiatric methods will be of no use. Some patients have been under psychiatric care for 10 to 20 years. They may hallucinate, speak intelligibly or not speak at all. Afraid to relate to others, they stay in their rooms. Also, thyroid disease is sometimes affecting children who do not want to go to school.

I have had experience with a number of cases in which symptoms of psychological instability quickly disappeared with heat treatment on the thyroid.

4. Parkinson's disease—This is not a norepinephrine-acetylcholine imbalance. Without a doubt, this is almost always associated with the thyroid. Too much acetylcholine is produced, so results may be quickly obtained by stimulating the sympathetic systems production of norepinephrine. Suddenly, the patient who could not move can write letters. Another who was shaking all the time can ride a bicycle.

Initial treatment with medicine yields good results, but the side effects are awful, especially later on.

5. Asthma—It may not seem related directly, but asthma also has a very close relationship to the thyroid gland. When heat is applied, there is almost always a very strong reaction over the thyroid. Asthma is considered a bronchial illness, but I believe nerves, spiritual illness and mental illness are involved. Often dust, hair, and pollen are considered the enemies of asthma. These influence asthma, but asthma itself is caused by an irregularity in the Autonomic Nervous System. If you balance the adrenal glands, thyroid and the vagus nerve with **ONNETSUKI**, there is such a good outcome. It is better not to use steroids. Of course, when one has difficulty breathing, it is difficult not to use medication, but one should not rely on it all the time.

6. Dwarfism is caused by the lack of growth hormone, which is caused by low levels of parathyroid hormone. I apply heat to the forehead area and nape of neck. This method is very effective with patients under 15 years of age. The effect diminishes with older patients. Be patient. It takes one year of treatment to see results. Fifty percent can be relieved or improved with heat treatment.

7. Autonomic Nervous System disorders—The patient does not feel good. They do not feel life working, have a light headache, feel a bit nauseous, and have joint pains and no appetite. Upon waking, he doesn't feel well and prefers to sleep during the day. All kinds of hospital tests will come out normal, but the patient knows something is wrong. These symptoms are caused by an Autonomic Nervous System imbalance. Menopause has similar symptoms and is also caused by a hormonal imbalance. Examinations with **ONNETSUKI** will definitely yield hot spots. Treat those spots. Check the thyroid. Hot spots will most likely be there too.

8. Infertility may be caused by many things. I believe it is related to the thyroid. A hormonal imbalance has affected the uterus and ovaries. In this case, you must balance every element. Women often become pregnant within two to three months after heat treatment is begun.

9. Irregular heartbeat, shortness of breath, difficulty breathing—These symptoms are often attributed to the heart and the patient is rushed by ambulance to the cardiologist. Most of the time, however, they come from the thyroid.

For example, I had one patient who thought he had a heart problem because of an irregular heartbeat. In the hospital, he was told to lose weight because the extra weight was straining his heart and causing the irregular beat. They forced him to go on a diet and fast. He could no longer walk and was in a wheelchair when I met him. He came to me because they wanted to perform heart surgery, which made him uneasy. My exam revealed very hot spots over the thyroid and around the neck. With my treatments, the heartbeat immediately calmed down. He was lucky not to have to undergo surgery.

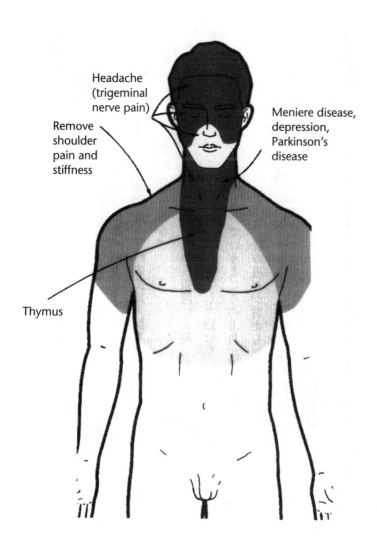

Headache
(trigeminal
nerve pain)

Remove
shoulder
pain and
stiffness

Meniere disease,
depression,
Parkinson's
disease

Thymus

THYROID A
(Meniere disease, headache, depression, Parkinson's disease 1)

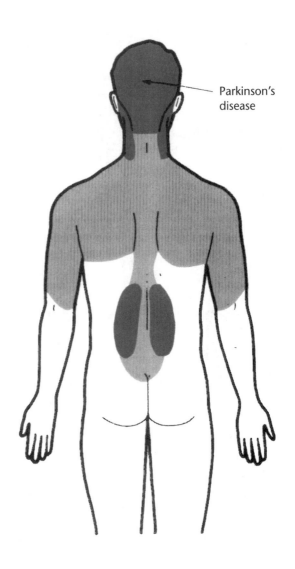

Parkinson's disease

THYROID A
(Meniere disease, headache, depression, Parkinson's disease 2)

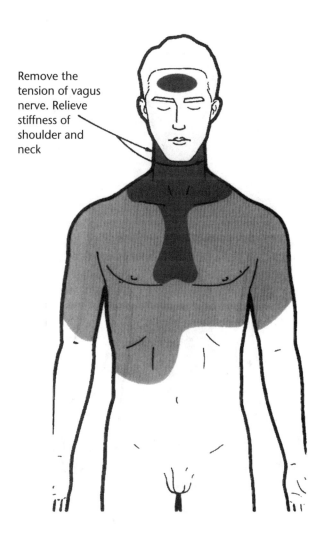

Remove the
tension of vagus
nerve. Relieve
stiffness of
shoulder and
neck

THYROID B
(Asthma 1)

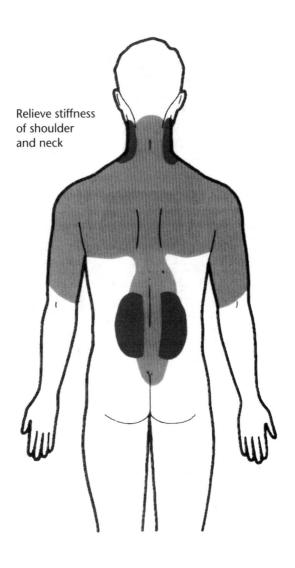

Relieve stiffness
of shoulder
and neck

THYROID B
(Asthma 2)

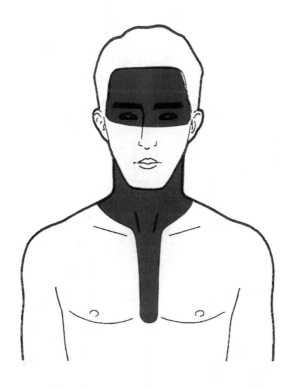

THYROID C
(Dwarfism 1)

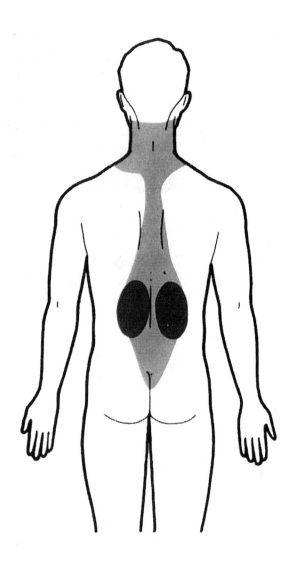

THYROID C
(Dwarfism 2)

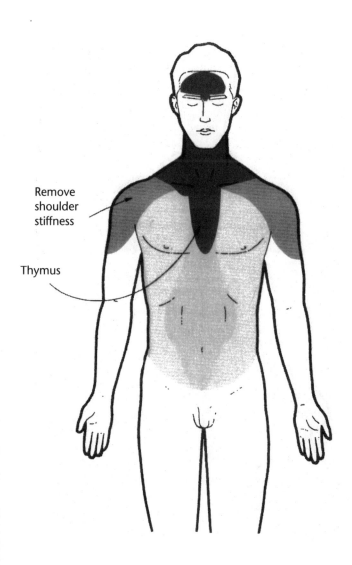

Remove
shoulder
stiffness

Thymus

THYROID D
(Autonomic nervous system disorder 1)

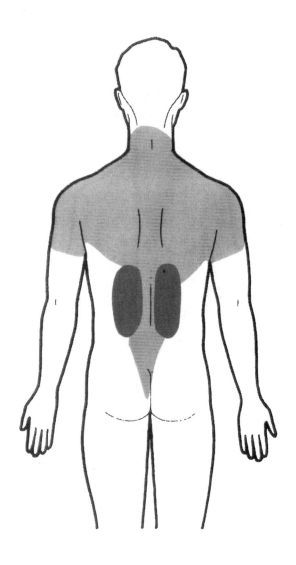

THYROID D
(Autonomic nervous system disorder 2)

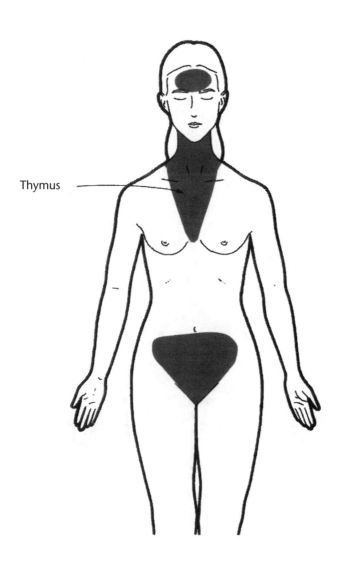

Thymus

THYROID E
(Infertility 1)

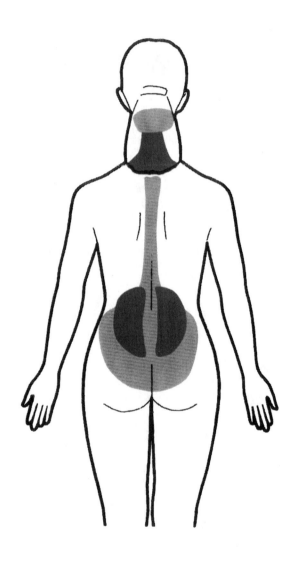

THYROID E
(Infertility 2)

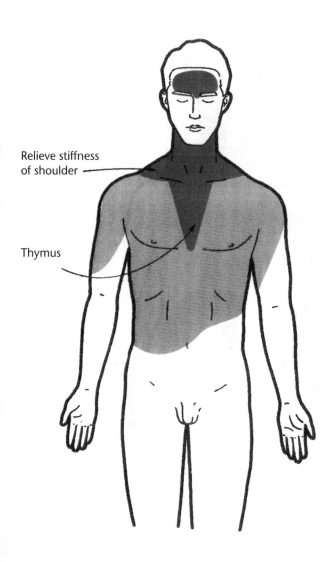

Relieve stiffness of shoulder

Thymus

THYROID F
(Palpitation, breath chokes, arrhythmia, dyspnea 1)

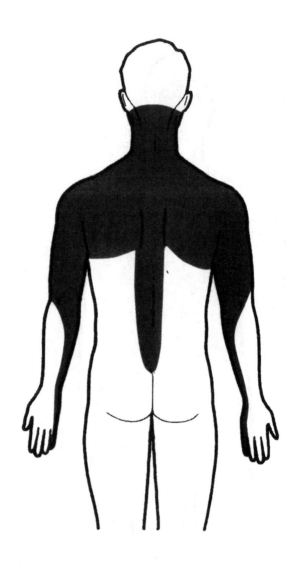

THYROID F
(Palpitation, breath chokes, arrhythmia, dyspnea 2)

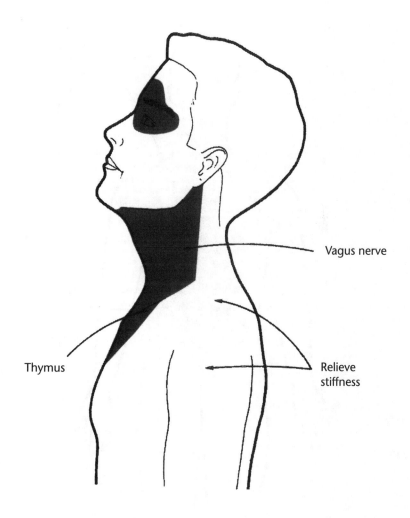

Vagus nerve

Thymus

Relieve stiffness

THYROID G
(Basedowis disease 1)

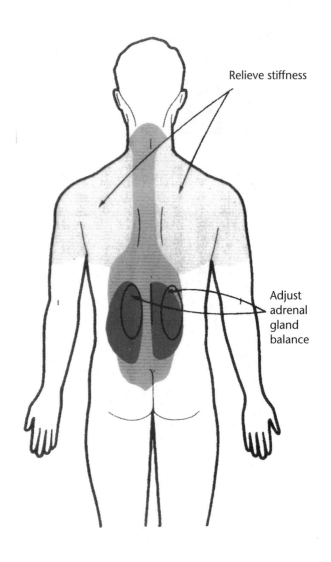

Relieve stiffness

Adjust adrenal gland balance

THYROID G
(Basedowis disease 2)

BLOOD PRESSURE

I believe there are too many misconceptions regarding blood pressure today. Each person has unique characteristics: shape, way of walking, and way of living. All of us are different. We are each a different animal. This must be accepted. Judging everyone according to the same blood pressure standard is very wrong. Some people are advised to take medicine to lower blood pressure without considering their size, etc. After taking this medicine unnecessary, gradually less blood goes into the brain, nourishment to the brain becomes less and less and the brain function, therefore, decreases. Stress, emotions and body fatigue also effect blood pressure. Thus, even in the same person, blood pressure varies. One may standardize blood pressure, of course, but it should be standardized on an individual basis. When one is healthy, blood pressure should be measured for many days and a standard reading should be derived from these measurements.

Blood pressure increases with stiff neck, arm, shoulder, and muscles, when one is angry or surprised, with strong desire, fighting and eagerness. Clothing, like tight brassieres, corsets, or bodysuits, can also increase blood pressure. Measurements should not be taken under these conditions.

If one has very high blood pressure, the first thing to do is to lie down quietly and calm down before taking medicine. If an illness is the source of high blood pressure, treat the illness, not the pressure. Using the heat method, the irregularity in the body is found and treated first. Later, the blood pressure is re-measured. No medication is taken.

ABNORMALITIES OF THE BONE

1. Osteonecrosis—This occurs as a secondary phenomenon of another disease. The top potion of the leg bone (femur), inside the joint space, is tight causing a lack of circulation and lack of nourishment to the bone. Right now, the treatment is a hip replacement surgery. One can emit heat around the muscles of this bone a number of times with **ONNETSUKI** to find hot spots. When circulation improves, the joint begins to heal. Therefore, this very difficult operation is avoided. If the operation were successful, all is fine. However, if it does not go well, the patient experiences difficulty walking. The heat method is successful most of the times. It does not hurt and treatment takes effect rapidly.

2. Disc herniation—Please see the section on Lower Back Pain.

3. Osteoarthritis—This is a joint disease, commonly affecting the knee. In its more advanced stages, the legs become "0" shaped and the knee joint swells requiring removal of fluid by a doctor. No matter how many times the fluid is removed, it comes back. When you bend the joint, it becomes very painful. You cannot sit Japanese-style. Many people undergo artificial knee replacement. Treatment with **ONNETSUKI** should be focused on the inner thigh muscles to stimulate the nerve, which travels into the middle of the knee joint. Often the swelling and pain disappears.

4. Whiplash—a condition which arises after trauma to the spine, for example, when one is in a car accident. The symptoms may appear immediately or many months-years later. Often people go to chiropractors forever for adjustments without improvement. There may be no irregularity on the X-ray either. some people become very depressed. Careful examination with **ONNETSUKI**

yields a hot spot in the area where the nerve was damaged due to the trauma. The chiropractic method of adjustments may not heal this, but through forcing change in the shape of the spine, it may worsen the condition.

5. The Frozen shoulder—In Japan, we call this "50-year-old shoulder." The arm may be moved, but is very painful. It worsens with lying down. You don't know where to put the arm to alleviate the pain. Any movement of the arm around the shoulder joint is very painful. This condition often occurs in athletic people, especially baseball pitchers, and housewives. For example, a baseball pitcher overuses the arm in a repetitive motion and at times cannot even move to throw the ball.

This type of shoulder pain is most often due to overuse of the muscles and the nerve is damaged. There are many muscles in the arm, so carefully examine with **ONNETSUKI** to find the damaged nerve and treat that area. Always keep the area warm (not cold). Do not use ice. Do not massage the area.

6. Traumatic spinal injury—This method can not cure a transection of the spinal cord. However, the following would be well treated in two to three sessions: spinal cord shock with paralysis below the waist. It is a temporary condition, lasting approximately two months and results in muscle thinning. The X-ray is not helpful. This often is seen in those who practice judo.

Heat treatment is tremendously effective for this numbness of the lower body. Look for hot spots along the spin and work in these areas for two to three sessions. Strong ligaments and bone very well protect the spine, therefore it rarely breaks or "goes out of alignment."

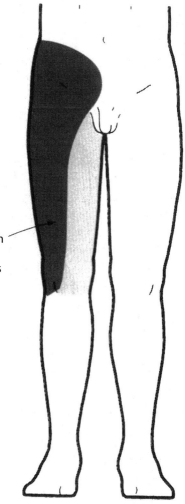

Use shiatsu and onnetsu together (left and right both sides, especially relieve the stiffness of quadriceps femoris muscles here)

OSTEONECROSIS A
(hip joint)

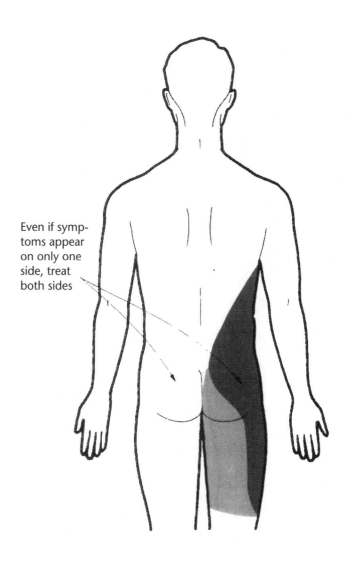

Even if symptoms appear on only one side, treat both sides

OSTEONECROSIS B
(hip joint)

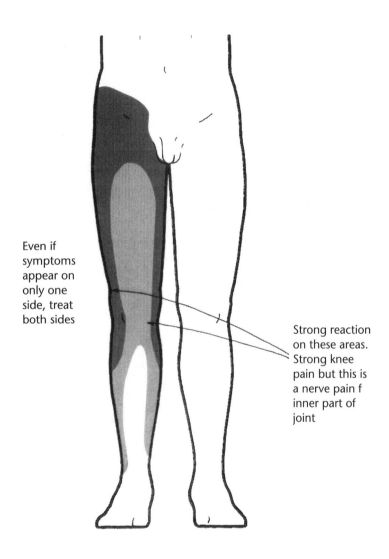

Even if symptoms appear on only one side, treat both sides

Strong reaction on these areas. Strong knee pain but this is a nerve pain f inner part of joint

DISC HERNIATION A

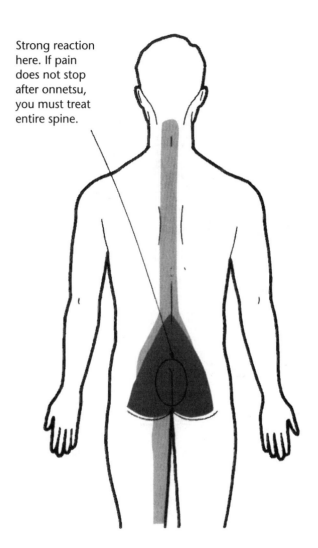

Strong reaction here. If pain does not stop after onnetsu, you must treat entire spine.

DISC HERNIATION B

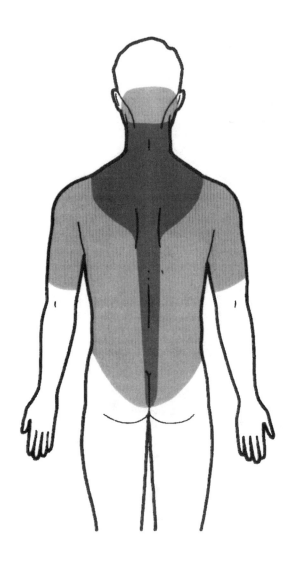

WHIPLASH

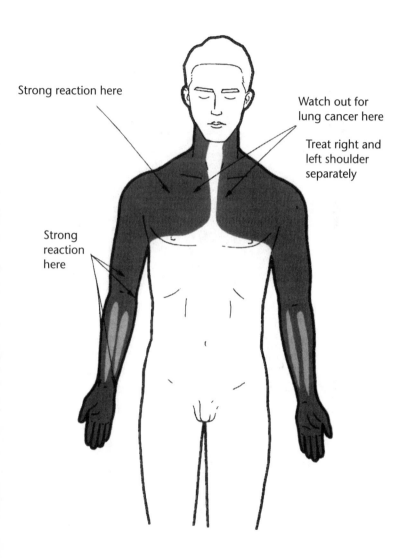

Strong reaction here

Watch out for
lung cancer here

Treat right and
left shoulder
separately

Strong
reaction
here

SHOULDER JOINT PAIN A
(frozen shoulder)

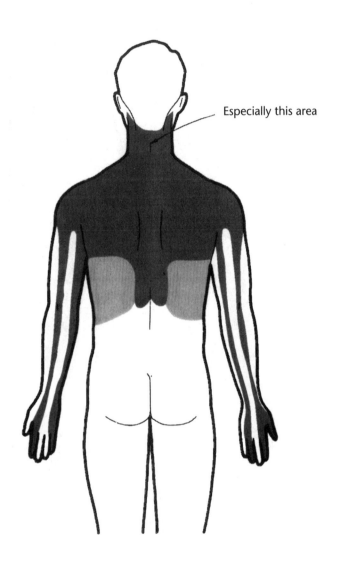

Especially this area

SHOULDER JOINT PAIN B
(frozen shoulder)

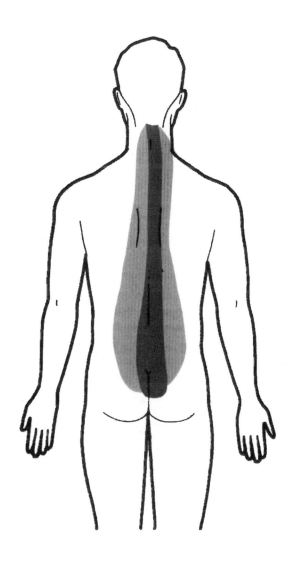

TRAUMATIC SPINAL INJURY
(mainly bruises)

NERVOUS SYSTEM DISEASE

1. Trigeminal neuralgia—The trigeminal nerve innervates most of the face. When it is injured, you get a tremendous headache. Sometimes, chronic headaches may be due to this. Three common causes are shoulder stiffness, fatigue, and thyroid abnormality. First loosen the muscles of the shoulder and then work on the neck.

Treatment:
    Do shiatsu on the triangle muscle of the shoulder and arm
        until they become soft and blood circulates well.
    Treat the thyroid.
    Diagnostic Pitfalls (see Chart on pg. 219):
    If A hurts, it may be misdiagnosed as a toothache.
    If B hurts, it is often misdiagnosed as sinusitis.
    If C hurts, it may be misdiagnosed as eye disease.
    These all are related to the trigeminal nerve and require
        treatment of the neck area. There is always a very hot
        spot in the neck.

2. Sciatica—There is tremendous pain from the buttock down the back of the thigh and also in the lower back. The knee area, front of the foot, and thumb may also be involved. When the big toe is affected, it may be misdiagnosed as gout.

The affected nerve, at the knee, separates to innervate the front and back of the leg. If the back nerves hurt, the Achilles tendon and heel will be affected. Placing heels on the ground can be terribly painful.

Treatment:

    The cause is spine weakness or irregularity, so examine from the nape of the neck down and look for hot spots. You have to be very patient and do this many times until the pain subsides.

    Try to apply the heat on the lower back, including the sacrum and tailbone.

    Apply heat from the buttocks to the sole of the foot and From the patella to the front of the foot.

3. Igoesntercostal nerve pain—The lower part of the ribcage and chest hurt, on one or both sides, with breathing. Sometimes, it is mistaken for angina or a heart attack. The pain may be under the armpit near the breast. When it is on the left side, it may be considered a stomach problem. The stomach should not be treated—this pain has nothing to do with the stomach.

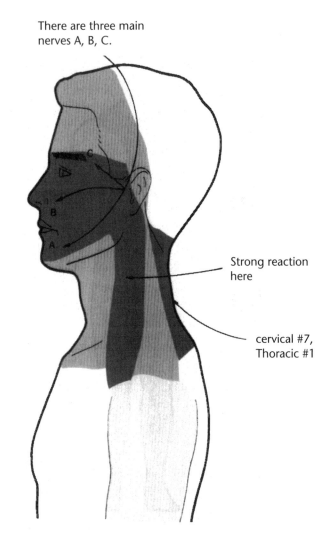

There are three main
nerves A, B, C.

Strong reaction
here

cervical #7,
Thoracic #1

NERVOUS SYSTEM PROBLEMS
TRIGEMINAL NERUALGIA

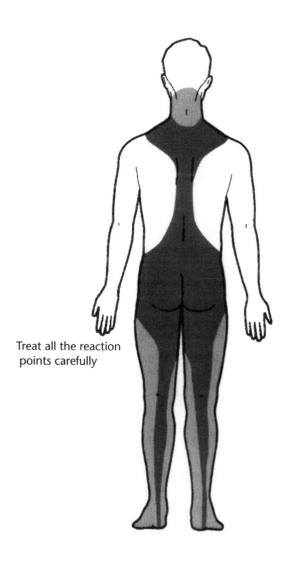

Treat all the reaction
points carefully

SCIATICA A

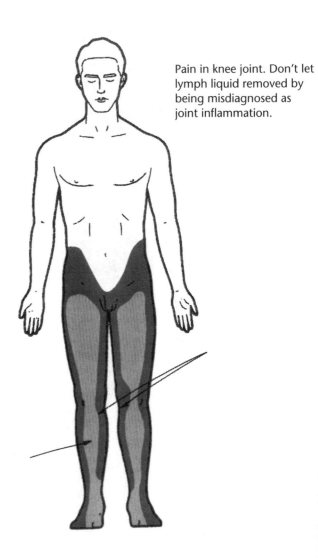

Pain in knee joint. Don't let lymph liquid removed by being misdiagnosed as joint inflammation.

SCIATICA B

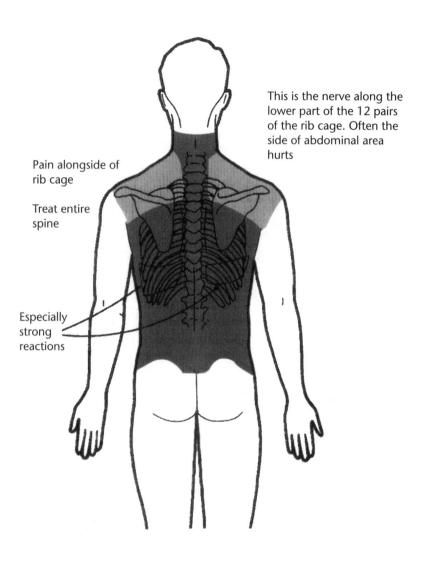

This is the nerve along the lower part of the 12 pairs of the rib cage. Often the side of abdominal area hurts

Pain alongside of rib cage

Treat entire spine

Especially strong reactions

INTERCOASTRAL NERVE PAIN A

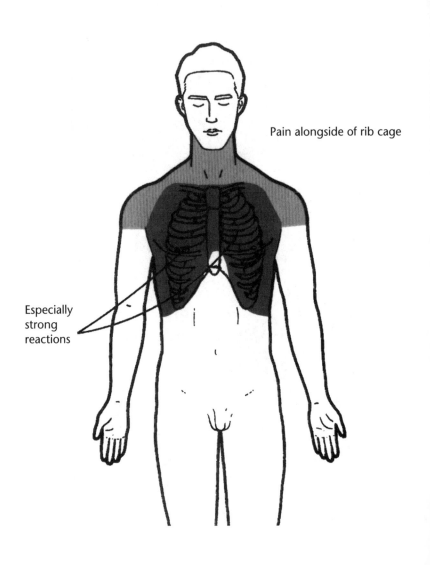

Pain alongside of rib cage

Especially strong reactions

INTERCOASTRAL NERVE PAIN B

LOWER BACK PAIN

Everyone suffers from lower back pain: it is the most common complaint. Nowadays, people do not walk much and are using cars all the time. Young people especially, have very weak lower backs because of their life style of driving cars all the time. It's dangerous.

There are many types and causes, not just disc herniation treated by a chiropractor. The first cause is muscle and nerve irregularity. In my opinion, the pain is not due to bones, but the associated nervous system and distorted musculature. The bone in the lumbar region is very strong and stable. It is like the middle pole of a tent. Therefore, if you attach the support ropes correctly, the middle pole remains stable. The ropes are like muscles that keep the pole straight. If you treat the surrounding muscles, the spin remains stable. Therefore, it is not the bone that should be treated but the muscle that is pulling the bone.

The second cause is related to the lower abdominal muscles. The back muscles and the abdominal muscles are like a seesaw: when one set is bending, the other set is stretching. Therefore, if the elasticity of the abdominal muscles is lost, then you will have back pain. It is important then to treat both the lower abdominal and back areas when there is lower back pain. If only the back muscles are treated, the lower back pain will become even worse and will not subside or heal.

The third cause of lower back pain is tightness of the lower scapular region. When this pulls upward, the lower back is strained.

The fourth cause is pulling from the leg and buttock muscles. When there is tightness in these areas, the lower back is strained with movement.

In all of these, adjustment is necessary. The body closely balances front and back, up and down, left and right. Do not only pay attention to local symptoms. With heat treatment, a person suffering with lower back pain for as long as three years can be healed in one week.

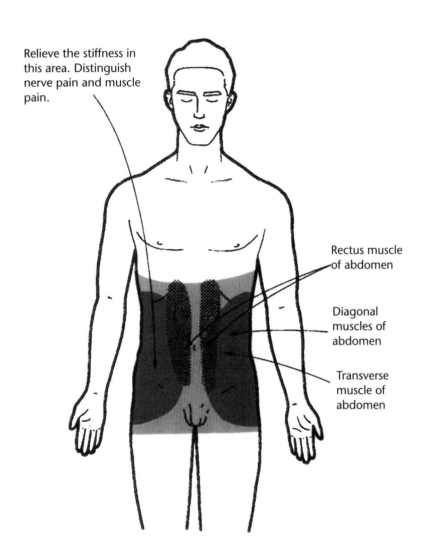

Relieve the stiffness in this area. Distinguish nerve pain and muscle pain.

Rectus muscle of abdomen

Diagonal muscles of abdomen

Transverse muscle of abdomen

LOWER BACK PAIN A

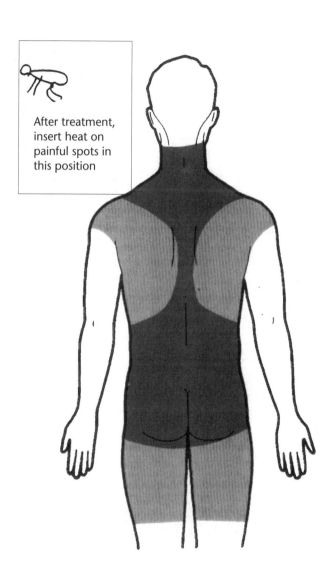

After treatment,
insert heat on
painful spots in
this position

LOWER BACK PAIN B

RHEUMATOID ARTHRITIS

From ancient times, this is one of the most common illnesses without effective treatment. Even to this day there is no cure. I think this condition arises from a hormonal imbalance. From my experience, not only is it the lack of adrenal hormone, but a total body hormonal imbalance. The fundamental treatment should be targeted toward achieving hormonal balance. This can be accomplished by restoring the Autonomic Nervous System to normal.

Avoid using pills to stop the pain. Not only they cause very bad side effects, but also healing becomes very slow and difficult. Patients with rheumatism can be very stubborn and difficult. Start the heat treatment and they will be treated very effectively.

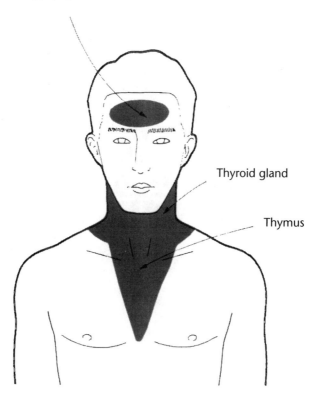

Hypophysis

Thyroid gland

Thymus

RHUEMATOID ARTHRITIS A

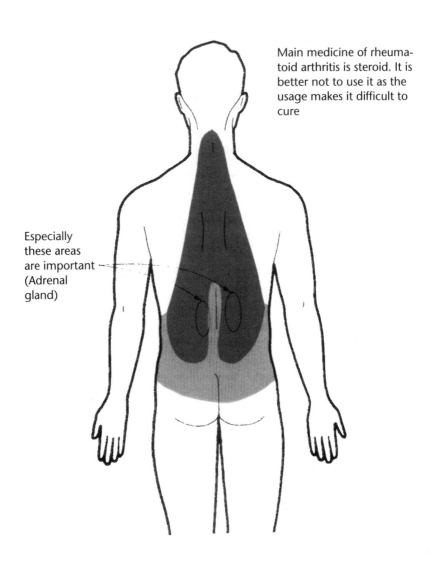

Main medicine of rheumatoid arthritis is steroid. It is better not to use it as the usage makes it difficult to cure

Especially these areas are important (Adrenal gland)

RHUEMATOID ARTHRITIS B

COMMON COLD

There are many symptoms of the cold and many causes of it. We say the cold is the first symptom of all disease. Often patients ask for medicine to cure the cold in one shot. Since there are many, many causes of the common cold, there is no such medicine. There is a way to avoid catching colds. One catches cold when the body is totally exhausted: days with hard schedules and much stress. In order to block stress from accumulating, do the heat treatment daily. It will help cure the cold with your own healing power and no medicines. This is easily done. By curing yourself, you develop the antibody for the cold. Do this method once with the help of **ONNETSUKI**. The next time you will not catch cold. Your own healing power is the one-shot medicine.

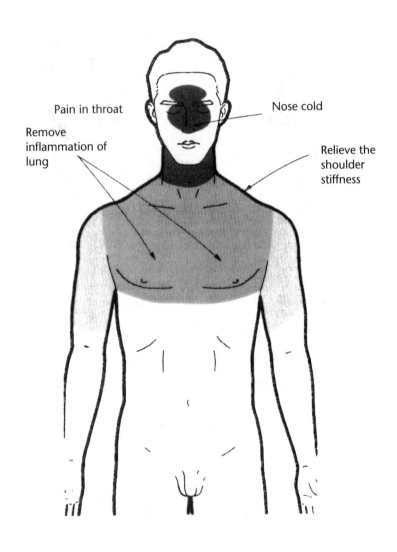

Pain in throat

Nose cold

Remove inflammation of lung

Relieve the shoulder stiffness

COMMON COLD A

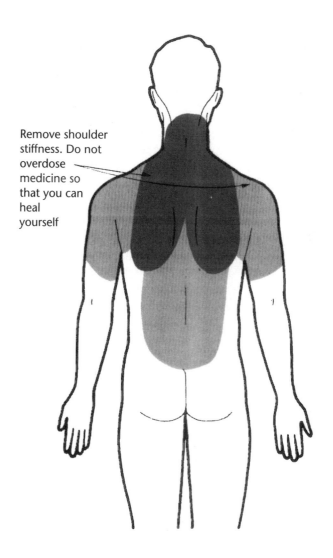

Remove shoulder
stiffness. Do not
overdose
medicine so
that you can
heal
yourself

COMMON COLD B

CLAUDICATION (PAIN IN THE LEGS DURING THE MIDDLE OF THE NIGHT)

This is a terrible pain in the leg muscle due to hardening. The muscles are overused and accumulate fatigue over a long time. A sudden move triggers tremors. Rigorous exercise, like jumping, may snap the Achilles tendon. The symptoms recur.

The pain is a result of "shrinking" of some of the thigh muscles suddenly, so they do not cooperate with other muscles. When you examine the muscles, you can feel the stiffness. Treatment should be in this area. The hard muscles, front and back, must be treated.

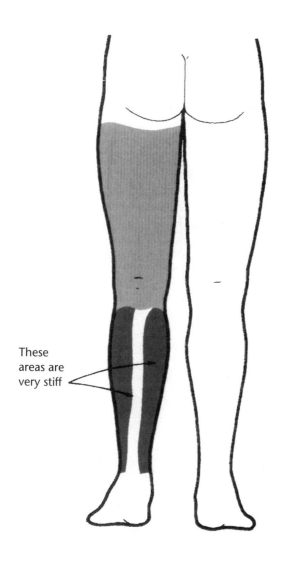

These
areas are
very stiff

<u>CLAUDICATION A</u>
(pain in the leg at night)

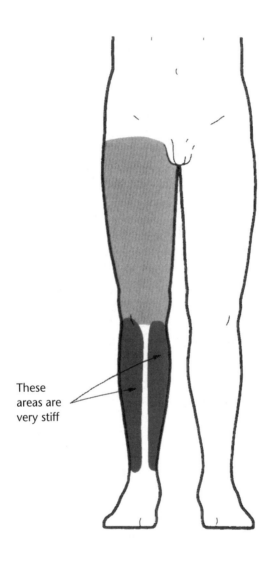

These
areas are
very stiff

CLAUDICATION B
(pain in the leg at night)

IMPOTENCE

This is a natural phenomenon of aging. From sixty years old, function decreases. However, it depends on the person. A 40 or 50-year-old could become impotent. On the other hand, I know an 80-year-old man who is sexually active. One's sex life does not have to end. The aging process will progress more quickly if one gives up. This condition is 95 percent treatable with the heat method and **ONNETSUKI**. In my experience, there was a depressed man, unable to marry because of impotence, which was healed in one minute.

Of course, the causes of impotence are numerous. Sex is often not completely understood. It is important to work with your partner on this matter, with compassion. Psychologically, a partner's kindness is very important. Also, a man should not think only of himself during the act. Consider the woman and how she should be treated—softly, full of love. Only insert when she is ready. The woman's discharge has many important roles—detoxification, pain reduction, and stimulator of man's excitement. The sex act should be different each time. Do not make it habitual and formalized. Study and learn much about the mystery of sex and enjoy the different tastes of sex. Ignorance may also lead to impotence.

Another cause is low levels of adrenal hormone. Medicine for high blood pressure can often affect the activity of the adrenal gland. Instability of the thyroid may lead to impotence. It happens after one recovers from an illness, of course, when the body is tired. Stress is also a great cause of impotence.

Treatment should be based on the cause. Men's and women's private areas should be handled with fingers. It is better not to use **ONNETSUKI** in these areas. The thyroid should be treated with **ONNETSUKI**.

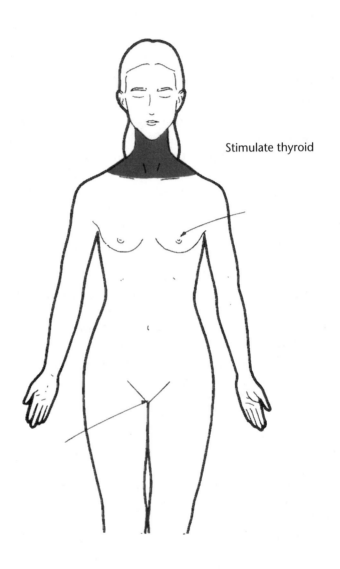

Stimulate thyroid

IMPOTENCE A

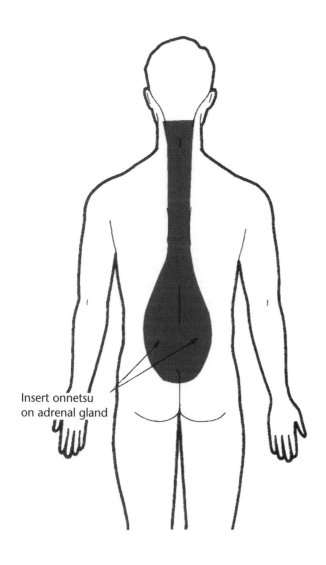

Insert onnetsu
on adrenal gland

IMPOTENCE B

STROKE

When this happens, treat immediately to avoid complications (i.e. paralysis).

Treatment:
The foundational treatment should be done very thoroughly.
The affected half of the head is very hot. Treat thoroughly until the reaction subsides.
The back of the sole should be treated very thoroughly.
Treat the entire body. Treatment within five hours of the stroke is very effective. But if more times lapses, there will be complications. If there is a delay of one week, the patient becomes paralyzed. Paralysis should be diligently treated for a couple of months and function will gradually return.
The patient should move as much as possible and try to live a normal life. Do not stay in bed all the time.

When unconscious, stimulate
this area with strong heat.

Do the fundamental
treatment thoroughly

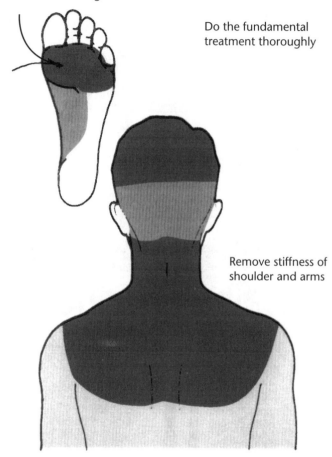

Remove stiffness of
shoulder and arms

<u>STROKE A</u>
(brain infraction)

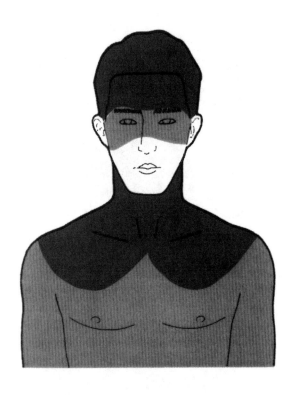

STROKE B
(brain infraction)

SPORT INJURIES

The training endured in order to become top-rated in sports is very rough on the body. Of course, the body is over-extended, the joints hurt, and knees swell. This heat method is very effective for these symptoms. I have treated sumo wrestlers successfully. The worst think one can do for these ailments is to allow the area to become cold. It opposes the healing treatment.

AIDS

This very difficult disease affecting the entire world has no cure and is becoming the prevalent illness of humankind. It is, of course, caused by a virus. I have only treated one AIDS patient. However, I feel all viruses can be killed because they become weak in the face of heat. So, I think AIDS can improve with the use of Far Infrared heat. I have not had enough experience with this. I would like to treat a number of AIDS cases. Also, I think we may find some hot spots.

INSECT BITES

Often insects carry and produce deadly toxins. These toxins may cause swelling. However, besides the affected area, the blood is also involved. Immediately apply **ONNETSUKI** to the bitten area. The toxins will disappear. Also, if one happens to travel with **ONNETSUKI** and is bitten by a snake, apply heat to the area and you will be helped.

Chapter 6

Testimonials

ACTUAL TREATMENT

WITHOUT EXCEPTION, INTERNAL BODY irregularities and illness reveal themselves as surface skin reactions during an examination with **ONNETSUKI**. One can detect any abnormality. Just apply **ONNETSUKI** and move it slowly on the skin. When there is some irregularity in an area around the underlying organ, the patient feels heat on the skin. Doctors say that internal illness cannot be diagnosed externally. You might think it is very mysterious, but I can diagnose externally, because I have paid attention to the relationship between the skin and inner organs. Even if there is some irregularity inside the bone, no matter how small, **ONNETSUKI** can find it. **ONNETSUKI** can even pinpoint problems inside the brain. Apply it to the top of the hair, skin skull, and eyes. An irregularity or sickness of the brain is noted clearly on the patients' skin. You also feel it in you hand. The damaged cells are recognized precisely: the area affected by the illness is especially hot. An area where nothing is wrong feels good and comfortable to the patient.

Also, it is much more accurate than very expensive machines. It's such a small, reasonably cheap machine, but it is very sensitive. Without fail, people are surprised. The examination in a hospital takes so much energy. With **ONNETSUKI**, you don't expend this energy and there is no suffering. The reaction is different depending on the illness and on the skin's strength. With benign disease, the patient feels slight pain or the feeling of having touched a hot iron. If the patient has cancer, even pea-sized, he feels a very, very sharp pain. The healer examines to find the area of abnormality and emits heat. Heat is continually emitted until the skin reaction disappears and begins feeling well. Then the illness has subsided.

When using **ONNETSUKI** for the first time, you may feel uneasy. It doesn't matter how strong the reaction is. It will eventually subside. It is like magic. A patient who gets better once is very pleased to find a hot spot to be treated. He may start to worry if there is no reaction. He is then asking even to increase the heat level. It is a really nice feeling.

Cancer is different. Some patients are in so much pain that they writhe, screaming and sweating. It is very different from reactions of other diseases, but it is the easiest to detect cancer from the surface. Sometimes, patients who don't have cancer are treated for cancer in the hospital. If one is treated for cancers by mistake, even if healthy, one may die within three years. It is like murder. This is a crime. This method tells you whether cancer is present or not. There is no misdiagnosis. You may be scared that you experience such a strong reaction, but be courageous. By the third or fourth treatment, this painful reaction will diminish. Keep doing the treatment and the reaction will subside. If you have the strongest reaction, the healing may be faster. No matter how strong the reaction is, when you finish the treatment, there is no pain. You can be active and have less pain. Patients with cancer up to the third stage can drive a car and lead a normal life. One may work and undergo this treatment at the same time. One will not die from Far Infrared heat, but will die from cancer. With this method, inner organ cancer heals quickly. After surgery, healing is slow because cells are damaged, **ONNETSUKI** helps faster recovery after surgery.

This chapter is dedicated to testimonials of actual patients who have benefited from this method.

Battling with Large Intestinal Cancer

— Misako Fukuyama from Tokyo

I became ill on October 4. At this time, there was some illness in our family and the relatives and I were under great stress daily. I had never been sick till that time.

I started feeling very strange sensations in the intestine. I was immediately diagnosed with intestinal cancer. I was admitted and had surgery. The surgery went well and I thought everything was fine. Then, I experienced diarrhea: up to 15 trips to the bathroom daily. Even when I went to the bathroom, I felt very strange—like something was left over.

A family member read about Dr. Mitsui in a dictionary on curing cancer. I left the hospital and started going to her healing center daily. I was very scared about my urge to go to the bathroom. After a few treatments, the diarrhea stopped. Mitsui found and diagnosed me with cancer of the lung, and treated it. There were no symptoms, which is usual because symptoms don't appear until the cancer is advanced. Three specialists in the hospital did not find anything in the lung, but Mitsui did.

Day by day, I became well. For those who have cancer surgery, don't take it lightly. You must try to fight, together with Dr. Mitsui and the Mitsui method.

Salcoydozis

— Kaoru Kawakubo from Tokyo

I am 36 years old and a mother of two children. Less than one year after the second child was born, I began losing vision in my left eye. I went to many hospitals for tests. They could give me no explanation. Finally, one hospital diagnosed me with SALCOIDOZIS. By that time, a chest X-ray showed many spots in my lungs. In my case, the nerve to the eye was affected. The doctors said there was no cure for this in the hospital—nothing could be done. We continued going to doctors for five years and nothing could be done.

Last fall, the doctors tested my heart and told me I had a heart disease. I fell into a deep depression, They gave me steroids and I got thinner. I was on the verge of death. I started taking ginseng, Maitake mushrooms etc. etc. I tried everything. They may have helped, but not fast enough for me. My body was getting weaker and weaker. That is when I learned about the Mitsui method.

Immediately, I bought the machine and saw the video. Instantly, I felt there was no other way than this. This is it. I can cure myself. I started going to Mitsui every week for treatment. I wanted to go everyday. I stopped going to the hospital because I felt so at ease when I was talking to Dr. Mitsui. She told me not to take steroids. Since last fall, twice a year I do a heart test. The day before the test, I always feel stress and have palpitations. After three months of seeing Dr. Mitsui regularly, I have stopped worrying and stopped taking steroids. I became well. The doctor was so surprised when I went for my heart test. I was so happy, I went to see Dr.Mitsui the next day and cried.

I have continued the healing treatment and have not had to have any more tests. I said goodbye to the doctor and the hospital. I believe wholly in Dr. Mitsui's method and in my healing power. Please, Dr. Mitsui, try to be strong and healthy forever so you may help everybody.

Breast and Lung Cancer

— *Tae Yonezawa from Hokkaido*

She had such confidence. Her statements were so strong and her kindness and compassion so great, I started to trust her very much. I received treatment for 5 consecutive days. Every time, the degree of pain reduced by about 20 percent. I felt things getting better. Up to that time, I had had a very aggressive cancer. I coughed abnormally.

My husband said that I sounded like I had lung cancer. The hospital tests came back negative for lung cancer, but Dr.Mitsui said I had it. She said that if it showed up on an X-ray, it was already very advanced. She treated me and within three days, this abnormal cough stopped. During the first treatment, when I felt such heat in the lung area and had such a strong cough, I thought the cancer was quite advanced . I am 68 years old. When I was taking a bath, I felt a lump in my breast. I went to the hospital where I was diagnosed with breast cancer. They operated on me right away. The cancer was in the second stage and I was told it would likely recur. It was all such a shock—mentally and physically. They tried to give me chemotherapy, but after hearing about the bad side effects, I refused. I was very uneasy if I had made the right decision. I was constantly very worried that the cancer would advance rapidly because I had refused chemotherapy. My husband reasoned that since we refused chemotherapy, we needed to think of other ways.

We read all the literature about cancer and studied everything. We read through about 50 alternative methods. The Mitsui method struck us by claiming cancer was very weak in the face of heat. I felt instinctively that this might be the right treatment for me. I also was doubtful that such a difficult disease could be treated with such a simple method. My husband and I decided to try it and went to Dr.Mitsui's institute.

The first day, I thought I would die from the pain. Dr.Mitsui assured me to bear it and not worry. I bit my teeth and endured. I was so surprised that the simple machine in her hand diagnosed the cancer and pinpointed exactly where it was. Dr. Mitsui even explained what stage it was and other characteristic treatments made my symptoms disappear. She said I had come to the right place at the right time. Within five days, I felt very strong and the cough completely stopped. I am very thankful.

I have seen many other people at the Mitsui institute get well. I also have seen two or three cases in which doctors had diagnosed stomach cancer and Dr.Mitsui said that they were wrong. I am very, very happy. This method can detect misdiagnosis because with *ONNETSUKI*, cancer cells act very differently than other diseased cells. I have been deeply moved watching her work with people without any desire for personal gain. Now I use *ONNETSUKI* twice a day on myself with good results. I am healthy and strong and work full-time. I also am trying to help others with *ONNETSUKI*. *ONNETSUKI* is my best friend. Thank you so much Dr. Mitsui.

Abdominal Area Illness

— *Yasumitsu Nakajima from Saga City*

My mother, 70-years old, has suffered with stomach problems for a long time. One day, she suddenly had incredible pain. At the hospital they told her it was fourth-stage cancer. I did not say anything to her. She had an operation but by that time the cancer was all over her body. They removed four-fifths of her stomach. The doctor said she would not last more than a month.

At the same time, I began having diarrhea and stomach pain when I had an empty stomach. Everyday, I lost weight. I was having a very difficult time. One day, by accident I read about Dr.Mitsui in a book. I went to her and asked for treatment. I explained about my mother and Dr.Mitsui asked why we agreed to surgery—we should have come to her first. During my treatment, the diarrhea stopped and my appetite returned. I was very surprised. I also had other problems—pain in my left arm that made it difficult to raise, and a few other unpleasant symptoms. The treatment cured all of them.

My mother came home 25 days after the operation. The doctor said she would just be home for a few days, but I stopped her medicine and started dietary healing. Also, I started to apply the heat method to her everyday. Gradually, the circulation came back. She had very nice color in her face and her appetite returned. She had had a back pain and a ringing in her ears all her life. Eighty percent of that disappeared. I know that her body is full of cancer, but as I apply the heat, day by day she looks and feels better. I apply it any place she has pains.

I am using the heat treatment for my stomach problem every day. I go to see Dr. Mitsui every month and this is keeping me very healthy.

Serious Rheumatoid Arthritis

— Kikue Fujitake from Chiba

My rheumatism started in February 1988. My hand and toes were very swollen and hard. I went to the hospital and was diagnosed with rheumatism. I was shocked and felt deeply depressed. I started to fight for my life against rheumatism. Everyday, I was in pain and crying.

I had gone to six or seven hospitals, to acupuncturists, to I could think of. I still have about 30 gold needles in my hand and toes. I tried alternative—herbs, hot springs, waters, diets. I did everything I could think of over the past six years. I have lived in pain daily. I couldn't get up out of bed. I would have to crawl to the toilet and then couldn't pull down my underwear. I cried all the time.

At the hospital, they gave me tons of medicine and I began to have stomach pain. I had to stop the gold needle treatment because of the side effects. My toes became deformed so that I couldn't wear regular shoes. Every second of my life was a fight with pain. I became very depressed and wanted to die because of the pain.

By accident, I heard that someone was doing heat treatment in Narita and that it was very effective with difficult disease and cancer. I pulled myself together and went to Dr.Mitsui. I really didn't believe she could do anything—because I had already done everything. I said that I would do her treatment so long as it didn't harm my body. While she was doing the treatment, she was talking and told me that rheumatism is caused by a hormonal imbalance. She reassured me that this treatment would stop the progression and pain. At first, I went once or twice a month. At the beginning it was so hot, I said I would never go back again. But every time I went, I felt much better the next day. With each treatment, there was less heat and less pain. Six months passed and winter came. Every winter for the past six years, I had suffered incredible agony. That year, I was fine. I was even going up and down stairs. A year passed and I was riding a bicycle. I could talk with friends and go on trips with them. It was unbelievable. Two years have passed and it is like a dream. I am well.

Now I treat myself everyday with **ONNETSUKI**, and once a month I go to Dr.Mitsui. My life has returned to normal and I am happy again.

Experiencing Dr. Mitsui's Method
— Masahiko Sudo from Miyagi

I am a 36-year-old businessman. For the longest time, I had a terrible, chronic headache and nausea. Sometimes, I couldn't do anything but suffer the pain. When I went to the hospital, they said it was a stiff neck and mental stress. They could find nothing wrong with me.

I heard about Mitsui from my boss and he took me to her. After 35 minutes of the first treatment, the heat became unbearable. Mitsui said that hot spots are bad places. Until then, I had taken pills when I had a headache. But with only one treatment, I stopped having headaches. It was like magic.

I had another illness. When I was 35 years old, suddenly I developed asthma and had attacks every time the seasons changed. I would go to the hospital for intravenous treatment. The doctor said there is no cure and I would have to learn to live with it. Mitsui said she could treat me two or three times and that I would be cured. I was puzzled, but I tried it. I received treatment twice and no longer have asthma.

My headaches, shoulder pain, and asthma have all been healed after just a few treatments. This is unbelievable. I believe in her words and methods. I have spent so much time and money going to doctors and hospitals. Mitsui's treatment took only two sessions. I am well now.

"I was a department store of illnesses"
— Keiko Oumi from Kanagawa

I am a 47-year-old mother of three university-aged children. I have spent my life raising three children and doing housework. It was like a war every day. Economically, it was also very difficult. I worked so hard trying to survive and raised three successful men in this society.

My body was exhausted. I had a stomach ulcer, gall stones, rheumatism. Menopause started and my hair started to fall out. Soon half of my hair was gone. I could not even work from the shame and pain. I had become a wholesaler of disease. The doctors said I needed to be admitted to the hospital, but I couldn't afford it. I had gone to a lot of health seminars on vitamins. I tried everything.

I had read and heard about *ONNETSUKI*, so I went to the institute. I started the treatment in September. By November, my hair started to grow back. This was such a pleasure for me. Suddenly the world became brighter because I stopped taking medicine. All the pains I had in my body have amazingly vanished. Stress from all these problems has disappeared too. As Dr. Mitsui says, our body has to have clean blood and "KI" energy running through smoothly. Then there is no disease. You need good nutrition and heat in the body. I am eating and drinking everything. I am very positive about life. As soon as I hear Mitsui's voice, I already begin to feel energy come through. Nowadays, I am only going every three months for a checkup. I am very well. If anything else happens, I will immediately go to Mitsui. I see in her clinics that everybody is positive. Even the cancer patients are laughing after treatment. I am completely healthy now and enjoying life.

Suffering from Severe Swelling of Abdomen

—Ichiro Maesako from Chiba

When I was 23, my appendix was removed. At 33, I was admitted to the hospital for intestinal blockage. The same thing happened when I was 38. The third time, while I was in the hospital, I read about Dr.Mitsui. She helped me tremendously.

Here is my story. After the removal of my appendix, I had constipation, bloating and difficulty passing gas. I went to many hospitals, including the one where I had the original operation. I went to acupuncturists and other alternative healers. It seemed to help a little bit, and the symptoms would come right back. I always was bloated and constipated. I had no control over my bowel function. I suffered so much. When I tried to stop the urge, my legs would tremble. When I heated my stomach a little bit, I felt a little better. My abdominal area was very hard to the touch, like a rock. In 1984, I couldn't even move. I sweated profusely and could barely speak. I called an ambulance and they could barely hear me. The doctors said that I did not heal well after the operation and that they could do nothing to help me. I lived like this for five years.

One day I went to the toilet and fainted. I was taken by ambulance to the hospital and was told the original operation caused the blockage. They said there was nothing they could do and that this could happen to 1-2 people out of 100. They said they could only give me painkillers. At that time, my wife read about Dr. Mitsui in a magazine. I went straight from the hospital to her institute. After that first treatment, in the car on the way home, I passed a large amount of gas with a loud sound. I had never heard anything like that. I went to her six times and became well. I could eat, drink and not worry constantly about the urge to go to the bathroom on the street

My Mother could not swallow any food and had lost all of her appetite. She was getting weaker by the day. I took her to Dr. Mitsui for treatment. She's also well now and we are both very happy.

Lung Cancer
— *Kayoko Ogawa from Osaka*

On November 24, I was walking the dog and suddenly could not breathe. I went to a cardiologist, who said I might have lung cancer. I went to a lung specialist and underwent all kinds of tests. I was diagnosed with third stage lung cancer. The tumor was in a difficult area to operate on. I had two chemotherapy sessions and radiotherapy. The cancer did not respond. Rapidly, I lost weight. I had no appetite. I vomited every day, but nothing came up. Of course, I lost my hair and my white cell count fell way down.

I lived with my 78-year-old mother and needed to take care of her. I didn't want to die. I started to read a book about alternative methods and found Dr. Mitsui. I checked into a hotel near the institute and went to Dr. Mitsui every day for one week. I was facing death so I was willing to bear any kind of heat or pain with her. I made all kinds of noise during treatment, but it wasn't serious. One will be saved. Do not think you will die. I found so much encouragement.

I had not been able to urinate, but after the first treatment, I returned to the hotel and needed to urinate. An unbelievable amount of urine came out. During the night, I urinated three times. I started to feel so good and began to have an appetite. My daughter, who was with me, was totally surprised. From the second treatment, the heat was more bearable and my chest was clearer. I started to eat three meals. The third time, during the treatment, I even felt almost sleepy. Mitsui said, "This was a good sign. You are saved." I came with such weakness and dramatically became healthy day by day.

My daughter was speechless. During the fourth treatment, I went on the scale and had gained two kilograms.

I even visited Tokyo. Before I returned to Osaka, I had detailed tests at the hospital in Tokyo. Everything was normal. My white cell count was 4,800 and my lungs were reportedly in good condition in only four treatments. I was so happy that I called Mitsui from the hospital. She told me not to be so relaxed about it. Cancer may recur, so one must do the heat treatment oneself all the time and go once in a while to the institute for follow-up. My husband is so happy. He said I could do anything I want. I am very happy and living strongly right now, playing the piano every day.

Stomach Cancer

— Koei Tanaka from Tokyo
I am a 35-year-old diagnosed with stomach cancer. First the doctors said it was an ulcer and then three years later they said it was stomach cancer. My doctor said that I needed an operation immediately. Then I would be okay. I did not want the operation. I learned about Dr. Mitsui's clinic and went to her. She told me that I did NOT have cancer and treated me. Since then, I have had no symptoms. I occasionally go to Dr. Mitsui to maintain my health.

Brain Tumor

— Kazuhisa Yamanoto from Yokohama
First, one of my kidneys swelled five times. The Hospital said it was a kidney cancer and operated to remove it. Next they said it was also a brain cancer and operated on the left side of my brain. Then they said that there was cancer again in the back of my brain. So I had another operation—four operations. Soon, they said there was another recurrence and another operation was necessary. I was very sick of operations and decided to do Mitsui's treatment. She gave me eight treatments before I went back to the hospital. They said the cancer was very small and had shrunk. I was very happy. I continued the heat treatments and am well today.

Breast and Esophageal Cancer

— Isao Kato from Tokyo
In 1989, they operated on my left breast to remove cancer. I am a man and breast cancer is very rare in men. Soon after the operation, I had difficulty in swallowing and felt something strange in my esophagus. I went to a hot spring, and I had hives.

I went to Dr.Mitsui. She said this was related to a duodenal block-age: the toxins could not pass through and were coming out on the surface of my skin as hives. Amazingly, with one treatment focused on the duodenum, the hives disappeared. Right now I'm treating the esophagus. It is going very well.

Intestinal Cancer

— *Tsuyoshi Nagano from Yokohama*

I had bloody stools. They said it was cancer located about 10 cm. from my anus. They told me I had to have surgery with anal recon-struction. I went to Dr.Mitsui for six or seven treatments. I also bought **ONNETSUKI** and treated myself. The lymph nodes and the throat also reacted and I received treatment in these areas as well. I am getting better. The reactions are all gone. Right now I am feeling much better and have no more symptoms.

Cancer of the Bladder

— *Shuichi Takizawa from Chiba*

I had blood in my urine. I could not go to the bathroom. I went to the hospital and was diagnosed with bladder cancer. Immediately, I had surgery and thought all was well. A year later, the cancer re-curred and I had another operation. When it recurred the third time, I did not want any more operations.

That when I went to Mitsui's institute. At first, I had unbelievable pain and sweating during treatment. After the second or third treat-ment, I stopped urinating blood and the pain during treatment less-ened. By the fourth time, the heat became rather comfortable and my whole body felt lighter. The pain I had experienced while uri-nating gradually disappeared also. Mitsui said I could eat anything I wanted. I was able to return to work. Mitsui told me that once you are operated on, you couldn't take it easy. Mitsui recommends treating with heat over surgery.

While I was getting the heat treatments, I received many calls, from all over the country, about cancer. I tell everybody Mitsui's rec-ommendation. There was an 80-year-old man with cancer of the bladder who was cured by Mitsui: he is now 91 and very healthy. Many people I know—with brain cancer, bladder cancer, esophageal cancer, and stomach cancer—have been helped. After 15 treatments, I have no more reactions to **ONNETSUKI**. I got to Mitsui twice a month for maintenance.

Water in my Ovaries

— Takiko Chiba from Miyagi

I was told my ovaries were swollen while I was in the hospital. Rather than surgery, I went to Mitsui for treatment. After 9 or 10 treatments, I returned to the hospital. I had no swelling and the doctors told me I was fine. An abnormality in the spine was also cleared. I am exercising and have a healthy appetite. Everyone says I look wonderful and have wonderful color in my face. They also say that I look younger. It's incredible. I do still go to Mitsui once in a while.

Abnormality of Thyroid, Kidney Inflammation, High Blood Pressures

— by Akinori Seno

When I was 16, I suddenly developed a rapid heartbeat and felt that my heart would burst. I had frequent urination, headache, and dizziness and felt cold in the lower part of my body. I always felt bad. The doctors said this was a thyroid problem and gave me medicine and shots. My blood pressure was high, and my heartbeat was fast even while lying down. I took herbal treatments, alternative medicines and fasted for 40 days. The headache and dizziness did not go away. I felt dizzy and my tongue and inside of mouth were numb. I couldn't talk normally. In the morning, upon waking, the symptoms were very severe. The tips of my toes and fingers were numb. I could not stand straight. My abdominal area was very hard and big. It felt as though my intestines were not working. I had horrible bad breath. I couldn't sleep. I was agitated and stressed out.

After the first treatment at Mitsui's clinic, my body felt very light. That night, I didn't go to the bathroom. I felt very well and slept well. The second time, she treated my thyroid area, which was very hot. After the third treatment, I felt so light and my headache stopped. I am well now and sleep deeply.

Asthma

— Keizo Umezu from Chiba

Since 1988, I had suffered from asthma. Every time the attack came, I would go to the hospital and get intravenous treatment. I had difficulty breathing and could not go to work. Suddenly, my breathing would stop and I would be taken to the hospital by ambulance. I had such an uneasy feeling that an attack could strike at any time. Every day, I was in a dark, deep depression.

Someone introduced me to Dr. Mitsui. During my first treatment, my breathing was very much at ease. I felt like the world was brighter. Mitsui said my face looked very different. At home, my family said I looked like a different person with a completely different face. I felt so hopeful. After two or three treatments, my breathing improved and my appetite came back. I am now just watching myself to make sure it does not recur.

Raynaud's Disease
— Sueko Tobe from Chiba
For seven years, I had severe pain in my fingers and toes. I could not even pick up the telephone. I went to many hospitals, but doctors could not find anything wrong with me. They only gave me painkillers. Gradually, these painkillers lost effectiveness.

That is when I went to Mitsui. This is one of the disease which the Japanese government has categorized as incurable "(nambyo)", but she said she could cure it if I would come two or three times a week. I went twice a week; six months later, I am completely cured. My hand is better. There is no pain whatsoever. They could not cure the disease in a big, famous hospital. I wonder how on earth she can cure this. I am most grateful.

Severe Backache
— Maiko Muroi from Tokyo
I have gone to Dr.Mitsui with lower back pain and leg pain. However, when I was receiving treatment, I had a huge reaction in my esophagus. Thinking back, I recalled having heartburn and an upset stomach. I worried about this, maybe it was the beginning of esophageal cancer. I felt so relieved that Mitsui found it. She told me that at that early stage it would not show up on X-ray and that a physical examination would also reveal nothing. It would have become serious later on. Treatment in the esophageal area cured my stomach and esophageal symptoms. I still do this therapy occasionally.

Healing Multiple Cancer with Mitsui's Methods
— Yasushi Fukuda from Tokyo
I did not expect much as I have gone through so much: Many hospitals, famous with cancer treatment, I even went to America. I first did not believe in alternative, holistic approach to cancers. But I was only waiting to die. I said to myself "I can not just depend on doctors. I must do something." I was diagnosed as having cancer in the

chest area, but that it was not possible to be operated on. I went through chemotherapy and radiation. My weight was down to 20kg from 62kg. I had terrible reactions to the Chemotherapy. Thinking America might have better treatment, I went to Hawaii, but was told in a Hawaii hospital that I will live a maximum of one month. I wanted to die in Japan so I came back. When I met Dr. Mitsui and told this story, she said "If you really want to live, it might take time, but you'll heal yourself". I almost argued with her saying "cancer is not that simple and easy" but I received the first treatment. I could hardly stand the indescribable pain. But, after the treatment, it was so strange, coughing subsided and pain was much reduced, after about 15 days, my symptom and pains were gradually gone. The test in September 1998 showed cancer has gone into submission. I am daily thankful for this treatment, and for my life-force energy.

Brain Tumors (Glioblastoma)
— A. S. N.   New York,NY

I have noticed remarkable changes since commencing far infrared therapy. The rashes are gone. The dangerously low lymphocyte _levels are advancing to the normal range. My body is no longer swollen. I have excessive amounts of energy, coupled with enthusiasm and a strong, positive will to create a new life for myself while helping others. My family and I are so grateful to Dr. Kazuko. Her persistence and dedication were decisive. She allowed me to imagine that I had a future, whereas other experts predicted a swift downfall. I will never forget.

Terminal Renal Cell Cancer
— P. D. V.   Plainfield, NJ

In April 2000, I was diagnosed with Stage IV renal cell cancer. I was told by my doctor that I had 5 percent chance of surviving the surgery, which I absolutely needed, or I would have no chance at all of living for more than a few days. The end of last year, a friend told me of Dr. Hillyer and Far Infrared treatments. Since December 2002, I have been receiving the Far Infrared treatments and I have stopped taking the injections. The quality of my life has remained excellent. At my last PET scan in February, my oncologist said the results showed that the disease was stable. I thank Dr. Hillyer and the Far Infrared treatments for helping to maintain my well-being and now I don't have to take in the injections any longer.

Glaucoma
— A. I.   Great Neck, NY

My first three sessions with her were quite intensive and painful. After my first six sessions, my eye pressure, which used to be 21, had come down to between 14 and 16. Six months later after I was diagnosed as having glaucoma, I was asked by my eye doctor to take a photo of optical nerve again. Six months ago, there were several numbers of red (3-4), which were "dangerous" and so were yellow ones, which were "quite dangerous". I had few green ones, which mean "normal". I still do not know what has exactly happened to me. Perhaps it is a combination of everything—meeting with Kazuko, receiving Shinkiko and *ONNETSU*, my colleague who helped me a great deal, my firm belief that it would be cured, taking Manda Koso, etc. I am also doing my best to be positive all the time.

Breast Cancer
— N. H.   New York, NY

I am a breast cancer patient diagnosed Stage IV with metastasis to liver and lung. After 4 days of therapy, my appetite began to return and my kidneys went back to normal. Six weeks later, I have no water weight, normal appetite and kidney function, and minimal symptoms from chemotherapy. My liver tests show much improved function and are almost normal. I have no cough and can take a full breath. I take no pain medication at all. I have plenty of energy. I can walk normally with no pain. Dr. Hillyer's therapy has saved my life and I expect to make a full recovery. I highly recommend this therapy to every cancer patient.

Loss of Hearing
— B.D.   Oakhurst, NJ

When one thinks of a dramatic happening in one's life, one generally associates it with a wedding, a birth, or a death in the family, or something similar. In my case, it was the return of the hearing in my right ear, since I have been unable to hear out of it for sixty-five years. All this dramatically changed when I attended a two-day workshop in New York City, given by Dr. Kazuko Tatsumura. In front of 10 fellow students at the workshop, I got my first personalized comprehensive treatment from her, in which she utilized *ONNET-SUKI*, along with added stimulation of some acupuncture points, plus the flow of her own personal energy mixed in. It was sheer magic, and *I was able to hear*, though faintly and with an echo; but the impossible was accomplished. I had my second treatment, and my hearing is still improving, and I believe it will continue. Words cannot begin to express my gratitude to Dr. Kazuko Tatsumura, who, besides being a gifted healer, is a wonderful human being.

Chronic Pain and Fatigue Illness
— *M. M. W.*   *New York, NY*

I have been ailing with a chronic pain and fatigue illness (fibromyalgia) for the past 10 years. Recently, I began FIR treatment with Dr. Hillyer and have been amazed that this treatment is effectively managing the pain, so that I no longer need to take medication for pain. I sincerely endorse this treatment as a way to manage pain without needing drug therapy, and ultimately as a treatment to bringing the body back to complete health.

CREST, Scleroderma, Rheumatoid Arthritis and Arthritis of the Spine
— *J. L.*   *Bayview, ID*

I have received the best news: Miracles do happen. I have gone into full remission, after ten years of being told "No, J., you will not heal, your disease is too complicated." Yes, this is the unthinkable, undreamable impossibility. I still do not dare to dream. I cried and cried when I was told I might be going into remission. Now it's a definite. I still can only believe one thousandth of this reality. I need to tell all other people with CREST, Scleroderma, RA, Cancer, any other *chronic illness or autoimmune disease* (about this **ONNETSU** –Shinkiko Therapy). It assists you to use your own healing powers. I will be more than happy to refer someone a treatment, answer questions, refer them to the closest available provider, or just to talk.

Skin Disease
— *M.R.R.*   *Bogotá Colombia*

It was a very special occasion that I will never forget because I hoped that you would give me a special treatment for my mother, which was supposed to be treated only by means of surgery, . . . She has recovered remarkably. Her skin does not scratch, we do not feel any swallowness, and she seems to be more alert than before. To make sure of our observations, we took her to two doctors: one is a general doctor ,and the other is the dermatologist (the doctor who was going to give her the surgery) who recommended us.

Both of them were very surprised when they saw how much she has recovered. They both agreed that there is a positive regression of the disease. I think this is a real miracle and I am sure the Lord put you in our path to help my mother recover and to give us peace and hope again.

Digestive Disease
— S. L. San Francisco, CA
My session was very helpful. My concern was my neck and my digestion. [Dr. Kazuko] was able to efficiently scan my body and discern that my stomach was dropped.She also explained that my neck pain was connected to the distress of my stomach. She worked on my stomach meridian, and she advised that I eat slowly, in small amounts, without any additional liquids. This is a problem that I have struggled with for years; it has caused me to be unable to digest my food and unable to carry a baby to term. I am most delighted with this new insight—it promises to be of great benefit in my life.

Knee Problem
— K. R. Chicago, IL
I've done much work to clear my brother's death, including five years of intense bodywork, but Kazuko was able to immediately intuit that I've been holding the sadness in my kidneys which directly related to my physical (knee) problems. She cleared that, as well as releasing a couple of knots in my neck and back, and I immediately felt my chest move forward and shoulders relax in a way like never before.

Respiratory, Allergies, and Digestive Disease
— G. S. Bellevue, WA
My two sessions with Kazuko had a very positive impact on my respiratory and digestive problems. My allergy symptoms and bloating in my stomach have disappeared. I felt very energized and relaxed after the treatments.

Conclusion

THIS BOOK REFLECTS 20 YEARS OF MY EXPERIENCE with healing. I would recommend this method of Far Infrared heat treatment for anything. It reduces pain and suffering as well as healthcare costs. I hope that this will help everyone to maintain health.

Someone else cannot cure sickness. You must know your body and you must guard your body. You must cure yourself. If you care your health on your own, you will not become seriously ill.

If you use **ONNETSUKI** Infrared heat even once in a while and treat hot spots you may find, you have nothing to fear. Even the scariest disease, cancer (which I do not view as scary at all), can be found at a very beginning stage and prevented from progressing.

You have plenty of Natural Healing Power in your body. The only thing you should do is to maintain or promote your Natural Healing Power every day. When you are sick, you know what it means to be healthy. Do this heat treatment before you feel sick, so that you can find the abnormality and treat it.

We have nothing in our bodies that are not necessary. Therefore, surgery should not be the first resort. The Holistic way of healing is so much better.. Cancer progresses without you knowing and by the time western techniques detect it, it is already quite advanced. The body is then hit hard by surgery, chemotherapy and radiation—three unbelievably harmful methods. Please you must try this **ONNET-SUKI** method before you agree to operation or chemotherapy. Even cancer is not an incurable disease.

About the Authors

LATE TOMEKO MITSUI (1915–2006) was born in Yamanashi Prefecture Japan. Graduated from Yamanashi teacher's college. For over thirty years Dr Mitsui devoted her life as an educator, and held many eminent positions in the academic field.

When she was 60 years old, she decided to make major career change to pursue her life-long interest of helping others and suffering people, and studied Eastern Medicine of all kinds. In 1988, she opened the Healing Clinic called SEIRYUDO.

She discovered that by helping to give extra energy (heat) into the body through certain area of skin, human's own healing power multiplied. She also recognized the power of Far InfraRed, and combined her Healing Method with this SUN'S natural wave of healing energy, established the Mitsui Method of Heat Healing. She helped numerous people suffering from diseases—especially with diseases that have no cure in Western medicine—and in the field of cancer, where her method has shown remarkable results.

KAZUKO TATSUMURA HILLYER, PhD, graduated from Toho Academy of Music, Boston University, New York University, and the International Academy of Education. She currently serves as director of Gaia Holistic Health Center and Okido Holistic Ltd. in New York, as well as directing the World Women Peace Foundation and World Religion Federation. Dr. Hillyer's numerous achievements and awards in the field of the arts, humanitarian work, and holistic health include the National Reputation Congressional Committee's 2003 Physician of the Year award; the Smetana Medal (Czechoslovakia); the Gold Medal of Cultural Merit (Austria); and recognition for "Specially Distinguished Services" (France). An internationally respected healer and educator, she lectures on health and spirituality and conducts seminars on a variety of topics around the world.